HELLO I WANT TO DIE PLEASE FIX ME

DEPRESSION IN THE FIRST PERSON

ANNA MEHLER PAPERNY

RANDOM HOUSE CANADA

PUBLISHED BY RANDOM HOUSE CANADA

www.penguinrandomhouse.ca

Random House Canada and colophon are registered trademarks.

Library and Archives Canada Cataloguing in Publication

Paperny, Anna Mehler, author
    Hello I want to die please fix me : depression in the
first person / Anna Mehler Paperny.

Issued in print and electronic formats.
ISBN 978-0-7352-7282-8
eBook ISBN 978-0-7352-7284-2

1. Paperny, Anna Mehler. 2. Paperny, Anna Mehler—Mental illness.
3. Mental health services—Canada. 4. Depressed persons—Mental health
Services—Canada. 5. Depressed persons—Medical care—Canada.
6. Depression, Mental—Treatment—Canada. 7. Journalists—Canada—
Biography. 8. Depressed persons—Canada—Biography. I. Title.

RA790.7.C3P363 2019   362.20971   C2018-902723-1
                                            C2018-902724-X

Text design by Jennifer Griffiths

Cover design and hand lettering by Jennifer Griffiths

Printed and bound in Canada

10 9 8 7 6 5 4 3 2 1

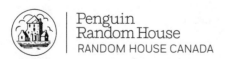

Penguin
Random House
RANDOM HOUSE CANADA

for Dr. Silveira

I myself am hell;
nobody's here—

—ROBERT LOWELL

Contents

HELLO I WANT
TO DIE PLEASE
FIX ME

Preface

How do you talk about trying to die? Haltingly, urgently: in messages and calls to friends. Abashedly: you stand in the middle of a hospital hallway on a parent's cell phone as your grandfather bellows, "No more stupid tricks!" Gingerly: you stand in your psych ward at the patients' landline, conscious of fellow patients watching TV just behind you, white corkscrew cord curled around your finger as you murmur to your grandmother who understands better than she should. Who is the first to tell you, as you lean against the orange-tinted counter with its row of cupboards for confiscated belongings below the sink, that you have to write all this down. And even though you put it off for months, agonize for years, you know she's right.

Quietly, desperately: in one medical appointment after another. Trepidatiously: to colleagues. Searchingly: in interviews. Increasingly loudly. In a book? With the world?

A disorder hijacks your life and becomes an obsession. Know thine enemy. Chart in minute detail the way it wrecks you and seek out every aliquot of information out there. Butt up against the constricting limits of human understanding, smash yourself against that wall and seek instead to map the contours of collective ignorance. Know the unknowns of thine enemy, learn them by heart. Because even if you never best it, never loosen its grip on your existence, at least your best attempt at understanding will give you some semblance of agency.

No one wants this crap illness that masquerades as personal failing. I had no desire to plumb its depths. The struggle to function leaves me little capacity to do so. But in the end I had no choice. I approached this enemy I barely believed in the only way I knew how: as a reporter. I took a topic about which I knew nothing and sought somehow to know everything. I talked to people in search of answers and mostly found more questions.

Personal experience has made me more invested in addressing the gross inequities depression exacerbates, in hammering home the human, societal, economic costs. The depth of depression's debilitation and our reprehensible failure to address it consume me because I'm there, spending days paralyzed and nights wracked because my meds aren't good enough. But this isn't some quixotic personal project that pertains to me and no one else. Depression affects everyone on the planet, directly or indirectly, in every possible sphere. Its very ubiquity robs it of sexiness but not urgency. I found this in every interview I did, in every article I read, in every attempt I made to sort out how the fuck this can be so bad and so badly unaddressed.

This book is also my way of exorcising endless guilt at having been so lucky—to have benefited from publicly funded inpatient and outpatient mental health care; to have maintained, for the most part, employment; to have had patches of insurance lighten the burden of paying for years of drugs. This shouldn't be the purview of the privileged but it is. We fail the most marginalized at every level, then wonder why they worsen.

I don't want to be the person writing this book. Don't want to be chewed up by despair so unremitting the only conceivable response is to write it. But I am. I write this because I need both life vest and anchor, because I need both to scream and to arm myself in the dark. Maybe you need to scream, to arm yourself, too.

PART I

IN THE FIRST PERSON

1
Cataclysm

What scares me most is what I don't remember.

And that's everything between scarfing sleeping pills on a Sunday night to waking fuzzily in the ICU days later, Velcro ties strapping my wrists and forearms to cold metal railings ringing the bed, keeping my erratic sedated writhing from disconnecting a maze of IVs plugged into my arteries. I discovered I was wearing a hospital gown and attached to a catheter (the latter, especially, not something you want to take you by surprise).

I was shocked when I surfaced at how much time had passed.

I've no recollection of the hours on dialysis. Just the lasting image of a churning strawberry-red slushee machine, which is how my dad described the lifesaving contraption days later.

I don't remember drinking antifreeze. Don't recall if it tasted acrid or cloying, its texture watery or viscous. The arresting electric blue I do recall vividly from staring at the family-size jug sitting under the sink every time I used the bathroom in the months after I bought it. (I've never owned a car.)

I can't remember conversations I had in the twelve-odd hours between the handful of zopiclone and the litre of antifreeze. But my text messages and call history betray me: I'd offered, in a near-blackout state, to rush out and cover a story that mercifully was taken on by someone else. When I asked about this later, the co-worker who called said I just sounded groggy. No kidding.

I can't remember being found in my apartment, overdosed on antifreeze, by two senior editors at *The Globe and Mail*, the newspaper where I worked at the time. Mortification overwhelms me each time I imagine the scene and I still wish I'd died rather than be found that way.

THAT, IN SEPTEMBER 2011, was my first suicide attempt, my first post-attempt hospitalization and my entry point into a labyrinthine psychiatric care system via the trapdoor of botched self-obliteration. For me it was an inexorable resolution—the only possible culmination of a conviction I'd had for months but kept putting off.

I was twenty-four and I'd just come off a pair of great assignments working as a staff reporter at my dream newspaper. But the preceding eighteen-odd months had been characterized by worsening, lengthening episodes of despair during which all I wanted was to die. For a while I could still immerse myself in my work, could still get that reporter's high, that bright weightless bubble filling my diaphragm as I chased a story. Could still convince myself, in giddy interludes, that my life had purpose.

But those interludes of story-chasing joy became spotty and infrequent, a radio signal subsumed by static. The bilious taste of failure swallowed everything.

THAT LATE-SEPTEMBER FRIDAY, two days before the attempt, I put the final edits into a political feature as sheets of rain thrummed against the wall-wide newsroom window. The nadir that in recent months had begun to engulf me at the end of every story's high was, this time, too deep to clamber out of. I felt scraped empty, nothing left and nowhere else to go.

I met family visiting from out of town for dinner that night at a fancy, poorly lit restaurant where if you drink enough silky-cold gin you don't notice how little actual food is exquisitely plated in front of you. I vaguely recall acting stupid-sentimental but not much else.

Stopping at the downtown Toronto office to pick up some things on my way home, I did what later felt like the first dumb thing. An acquaintance—someone I'd met once who had subsequently added me on Facebook and with whom I'd exchanged muted messages during periods of mutual insomnia—struck up the most casual of "how you doing" online conversations. To which I responded that I was finally going to kill myself.

Ha ha, not funny
Not joking
Don't kill yourself
But I want to

The exchange ended with my saying I probably wouldn't do anything. Anyway, g'night. Talk to you later. I think this is when I deleted my social media accounts.

I wouldn't have said anything to Facebook Guy in the first place were it not for the tenuousness of our acquaintance and the atonality of online conversation, which left me feeling fairly confident he wouldn't do anything.

Wrong. Wrong on all counts.

I didn't kill myself that night. Didn't even try. Crashing hard from serial work weeks without weekends and a boozy family dinner, I collapsed in my apartment, fell into zonked sleep fully dressed on an unmade bed.

The second dumb thing was missing the incessant calls to my phone, left on vibrate. This poor dude I barely knew panicked. He contacted a mutual friend, who called me, then the police. It was their call that I finally surfaced from slumber to register. I was just out of it enough to see the blocked number and irrationally assume it was the desk—my editors—calling in the middle of the night with some urgent query or request. Workaholic reflexes overrode my desire to be eternally alone.

Instead it was a police officer wanting my address and I, in sleepy half-stupor, gave it to him. Except then, of course, they came to my apartment.

I didn't know how you're supposed to respond when a pair of cops shows up at your door at three o'clock in the morning saying they've been sent because someone told them you're trying to off yourself. The keenest emotion I recall was embarrassment.

"The place is a mess," I apologized.

That was an understatement. I've never been neat but the conditions of my ground-floor apartment in a shabbily aging building with a mouse problem compounded by my own apathy were probably startling. In my defence, the hole in one kitchen wall leading straight outside, the mildewed bathroom ceiling, the missing bathroom tiles where sink met floor, the warped wood floorboards that seemed impossible to clean, were not my fault; they predated me. I just hadn't mustered the will to have them fixed. The overall disarray, the papers everywhere, the food wrappers and containers, the sticky mousetraps in need of chucking, all contributing to the overall thick atmosphere of must that had crescendoed over the preceding months—that was my bad.

"It's okay," one officer said. "We're used to messes."

But there was something in this mess or in my bleary "everything's fine" mumblings that convinced them I should not be left alone. They didn't cart me away or cuff me but when I asked if I could stay home and go back to bed, the answer was firmly negative. So I went with them, unwilling; their force implicit, not physical.

I wondered only later how that scene would have played out had I been Black and male, and what would have happened if I had simply refused to go.

That was my first ride in the back of a cop car, a barrier between me and the front seats. It was a short trip to the nearest hospital, where the three of us sat in the dull beige fluorescence of the ER waiting room and made small talk until someone arrived to usher me into the psychiatric crisis ward at St. Joseph's Health Centre—St. Joe's, as its familiars call it. We somehow—reporter reflex—started talking about their careers. One of the officers had been a sound technician in another life and I made a mental note to pass the name of his program to a kid I'd interviewed days earlier who wanted to study music production after finishing high school.

They were decent guys. They must've been all too accustomed to dealing with situations like mine, with people more erratic and less cooperative than I. My situation—despondent suicidal chick in an apartment given over to entropy—was a breeze compared to nightmare scenarios of agitated, sick, harmless people killed by police in hospital gowns,[1] on streetcars,[2] in their own homes or apartment buildings.[3] These cops just talked to me until they were free to go back to their jobs, catch some bad guys. Given that some cops spend hours effectively babysitting someone until a hospital can deal with them, they were no doubt relieved when I was led away into the crisis ward and became someone else's responsibility.

If you're ever picked up by police and carted off to hospital in the middle of the night, I recommend bringing a warm sweater and a good book (cell, charger, wallet, writing implements and health card are also worthwhile accessories). I, short-sighted fool, was wearing the previous day's skirt, a T-shirt and a thin raincoat I'd grabbed groggily on the way to the police cruiser so I'd have a pocket for my keys, which were quickly confiscated along with my phone, pen and the digital recorder still in my jacket pocket from work, a day and a lifetime earlier.

The crisis ward was dark and bare and cold and I was bored out of my mind. Curled up shivering on a plasticky hospital chair, grimly suicidal, I mentally cursed Facebook Dude for freaking out when clearly—I told myself as I brooded on death—I hadn't been serious. Kicked myself for caving to the desire for human contact and then not even bothering to try to follow through on my own death.

I was almost demented with fatigue. I remember someone offering me a bed, which I declined—afraid that acquiescing would mark me a patient, someone who belonged there, no different from the bedridden man quietly moaning behind me. I didn't belong, I told myself. I just needed to clear up this misunderstanding.

A young kid—fourteen, maybe—regained consciousness in an adjoining room. The orderly returning his backpack had to explain to him how he'd wound up there after police found him unconscious and alcohol-poisoned at a friend's house party. For the next six hours I sat there envying his escape. The blessed orderly took pity on me when the paper arrived; I've never been so glad to see the flyer-filled Saturday *Star*. By the time a tired-eyed psychiatrist saw me around nine o'clock I would have said anything to get out of there so as to kill myself as soon as possible.

It became immediately clear she had no idea I'd been brought to the hospital's psychiatric crisis ward in a cop car, against my will: when I said I didn't want therapy, just wanted to go home (with some pills to help me sleep, please), she gave me a withering-pitying look as if to ask why I was wasting her time. By ten o'clock I was out in the sharp bright morning making a beeline for a pharmacy to fill a disappointingly small prescription for the sleeping pill zopiclone. (I've never needed chemical help falling asleep.)

The rest of Saturday was strange. I think I slept. I think I tried to go for a run along the lake but couldn't muster much energy, run-walking and petering out about a kilometre from my apartment, on a rocky outcropping on the Etobicoke side of the Humber Bridge. Pacing the rocks, I exchanged a surreal series of short emails with a colleague who'd heard about my night in the crisis ward and was tentatively trying, it seemed, to make sure I was okay without becoming embroiled in whatever weird life drama I had going on. Accustomed as we've become to communicating textually, I can tell you there are times when hearing someone's voice—as anxiety-inducing and time-consuming as that can be for the caller—would make a big difference.

I knew better now than to say how I felt. "I'm fine. Really. Don't worry."

I think I would have tried to kill myself that night were it not for an unexpected Sunday assignment, a campaign budget announcement for which I felt obliged to stay alive. I remember astonishing watery sunlight and cold wind whipping wet hair against my face as I biked downtown Sunday morning. I negotiated the incongruous banality of a technical briefing in a windowless hotel conference room. I remember joking with a fellow journo about our lack of math skills. There was a scrum: something about provincial debt, something about early voting; a web file that needed updating and contextualizing; counter-claims from opposing parties to parse and write up.[4] Then I was free.

I think I bought groceries and the Sunday *New York Times*. I think I loitered over tea and wi-fi in a Queen Street café-bar. Eventually I made my way home. It was past midnight by the time I grabbed the plastic jug of bright-blue antifreeze from its spot in the bathroom, poured it into a pair of oversized pottery mugs. (Suicidality notwithstanding, I wasn't about to chug antifreeze from the jug: I had standards.) I placed the mugs of poison on the floor beside my burgundy futon-couch. I recall keeping the newspaper fanned out in sections beside me. Why? As a prop? Did suicide seem less pathetic if I just pretended I was catching up on world news?

I swallowed the fistful of pills first, waited expectantly. I remember registering disappointment in their inefficacy before consciousness and memory dropped off a cliff.

2

When You Try to Die and Don't

Monday would have been when those unnerving ghost-exchanges took place, when I spoke with a colleague about who would cover an electoral spat over cancelled gas plants. So it must have been shortly afterward that I swallowed the antifreeze. I think. I don't know. So terrifyingly blank is that space in my memory that anything could have happened to fill it. I only insert the most likely chain of events in the hope that if I repeat it enough the repetition will confer an internal sheen of truth.

I do know it wasn't until Tuesday that my unresponsiveness began to worry people. Following a series of phone calls and emails between co-workers and friends wondering where I was, a pair of senior editors from work arrived at my building just as, separately, my friend Wesley did. Wesley knew me. He'd seen me at my less-than-best. But the editors? Intimidatingly smart and really not the kind of people you'd expect at someone's sickbed, these two managers held my career in their hands. I wouldn't want them to see me fumbling through a fruitless phoner, let alone mid-methanol overdose.

Truth is, they saved my life. But the shame and self-revulsion I feel at the thought of being found there by them hasn't gone away.

They got into my apartment (Had I left the door open? Why?) and found a mess.

The place was a mess. I was a mess, covered in my own puke. It pained me to be told, months later, that I wasn't totally unconscious—just not terribly responsive or remotely cogent. They called the police and tried to figure out what I'd taken. They failed: it wasn't until my cousin and dad were dispatched later that week to brave the premises that they found the open antifreeze container, about a quarter of the four-litre vessel gone.

Police arrived first, then an ambulance. I'm told I joked with paramedics while being wheeled out on a stretcher. What stands out for my friend Wesley, poor bastard, is how filthy my kitchen sink was. He and one of the editors followed the ambulance to St. Joe's feeling there was little they could do right then apart from figure out who needed to know what. He and a group of five close friends—the people who became my rocks in the weeks and years following—then huddled to discuss what to do. Among other things they asked each other how emotionally invested they were each prepared to become in this. Surely most people in their right minds would go running in the opposite direction. I don't know why these people didn't disappear. (Other friends and colleagues did. I don't blame them.) I don't know why they decided to subject themselves and their own challenging lives to my prickly, unwelcoming, messy state of affairs. I don't know whether they've regretted it. I've lacked the guts to ask. But my god, I'm glad they did.

WHEN I SURFACED my parents were there. My poor parents, who had flown in from Vancouver, who had by then had about thirty-six hours to acclimatize to the idea—and the sight—of their daughter hospitalized after a botched suicide.

Years later my mom recalls being regarded by the kidney specialist who had come to oversee my treatment. "She said, 'You're so calm.' And I realized I just had kind of been so focused on fixing it. Get here, fix it. I couldn't really entertain the alternative."

One of the first things mental health practitioners tell you after you try to die is that your recent attempt is not selfish, not a misery you've inflicted on those you love most, but a fatal final symptom of a disease that's destroying you. Which, sure. Fine. But seeing my younger brother's face in that psych ward after he'd flown in from his first weeks of law school convinced me I deserved to die in the most torturous way imaginable. Loving people so much it hurts doesn't necessarily negate the need to die; it just makes you hate yourself more for all the pain you cause, makes you feel your death would be a gift.

Recollections return in uneven swatches. Sleeping pills, even when taken as directed and not downed like peanuts, are one hell of an amnestic. Now, when I try to pull memories forward from mental recesses for reinspection, I find them frayed and moth-munched, viewed through a lens messily smeared with Vaseline. Some reappear in high definition much later: the way I tried to read a book in my ICU bed only to find the words bounce as my squinted eyes stung and watered, unfocused.

"This is a shitty book," my mom claims I said.

I owe Patrick deWitt an apology: I can't look at the original cover of *The Sisters Brothers* without a shuddering flashback to the pain behind my eyes, the panic of being unable to read. This in all likeli-hood was an after-effect of the antifreeze, which, if it doesn't kill you, can make you permanently blind. This inability to comprehend the written word was mercifully short-lived; I don't know how I'd have coped otherwise, thus disoriented and unmoored.

AFTER TWO OR THREE days in the ICU they put me in the short-term psych ward. I toddled over in that sky-blue dignity-depriving hospital gown, changing in the bathroom into civilian attire. The psych ward had no windows and no privacy, just beds separated by curtains sliding on rods.

I was so out of it when first ushered in from the ICU that nothing registered. Surely I'd leave soon. Surely I'd be back at work in no time. A return to the newsroom that centred my universe was all

I needed, I told myself. Find a way out. Everything will return to normal.

Or not. There were Forms to contend with. I had just become one of a growing number of psych patients kept in hospital against their will—I was put on a Form formalizing my committal by a doctor deeming me too crazy to make my own decisions.

Every jurisdiction in Canada, the US and much of Europe still has some kind of medical-legal framework for dealing with people who lack insight into their conditions or lack the capacity to make decisions. You can put someone in hospital against her will if a doctor decides—sometimes at the urging of police, a judge or family members—that she's in danger of causing imminent harm to someone, including herself. (Important to note: she still has rights when you do this, and when you take away some rights, protecting the others becomes more important than ever. More on that later.) In Ontario,[1] where I live, it begins with a Form 1,[2] which subjects you to a seventy-two-hour "hold" that allows for a psychiatric assessment. By the time I toddled into the short-term psych ward, the seventy-two-hour hold that I'd been placed on in the ICU had just about run out, necessitating a new one: a Form 3 this time,[3] which allowed me to be kept against my will for two weeks. I was too out of it to know this and nobody told me until days later, giving me the sinking feeling of being suddenly trapped.

There are two primary reasons why you'd be upgraded to a Form 3. One is that you're incapable of consenting to treatment but you've been treated and got somewhat better before and they have reason to believe, based on that prior experience, that you really need that treatment now or your condition will seriously deteriorate. But "deterioration" is pretty broad and subjective. So that significantly increases the pool of people eligible for involuntary hospitalization—which is either a boon to patient health or a draconian way to lock more people in hospital, depending whom you ask.

The other reason, my reason, is that they're fairly certain you have a mental disorder and there's a serious risk of someone getting seriously hurt or impaired. It has two key sub-categories: "Bodily harm to the patient" and "Bodily harm to another person." The seeming fungibility of that check-mark differentiation—Does this crazy person pose a threat to herself or to other people? Should I be scared for her, or of her?—is what freaks out so many when it comes to people with mental illness. It's what tormented me at the time, certified by that form, even with the "harm to others" box unchecked.

Some assume people with mental illness are going to kill them, or attack them, or commit some horribly violent, depraved act without warning or reason. We assume this despite centuries of evidence to the contrary. People with mental illness are far more likely to be victims of violence than its perpetrators.[4] When they get the treatment they need they're highly unlikely to hurt anyone.

I thought I understood that. Until I realized, that day in that hospital, how scared I became of myself. No one checked off that "danger to others" box on my form. Only the "danger to self." But the two boxes are so close together! Just its paperwork proximity was enough to convince me I posed a threat without even realizing it. Was I going to hurt people against my inclination? Was I a murder-suicide risk? No, my doctor would emphatically tell me in the months following. Of course not. But unconscious biases run deep, and this wracked me for a while.

But in the immediate term, this crazy-person paperwork meant I couldn't leave the hospital. I couldn't leave the ward without an eagle-eyed escort. I couldn't shave. I couldn't charge my recently returned cell phone without supervision. I entered a bad *Groundhog Day* remake. Over the course of five-ish days in the short-term ward, I murmured the same thing in the same chastened tone to an endless parade of health care workers armed with clipboards: a slim nurse with an eyebrow ring, not much older than I was; an affable social worker; another nurse who told me about his wife and their efforts to have kids and who remembered me, years later, when I was back as an outpatient; the staff psychiatrist who was there less often but who, when she was, was clearly in charge.

I repeated it sitting on my bed, dutifully completing my daily suicidality checklist: "It was a one-off." I repeated it sitting on the almost-comfortable couch of the glassed-off rug-floored consult room ("I thought I wanted to die because I thought I felt hopeless. I don't feel that way anymore.") I repeated it crouched by the low coffee table laden with coping-strategy worksheets and dated magazines in the common area ("It was such a dumb thing to do. I realize that now. I wish I hadn't done it. I won't do it again."). I repeated it so much I believed it myself.

So much for my model-patient alibi. What do you tell the people you love about the thing you did that caused them pain? You have abashed phone conversations with your Calgarian grandparents. You lie to your aunt when she makes you promise you'll never try again. You hold your breath and avoid the topic altogether. My mother's mom, the Los Angelina Auschwitz survivor and the strongest nonagenarian you've ever met, I've never told, although my mom told her years later, a harrowing impulsive disclosure and a brutalizing thing for her to hear. She's ninety-three and I still feel ashamed just talking to her, the epitome of life's triumph against all odds, having expended so much time and effort and brainpower toward my own death.

From the moment of my arrival at the crisis ward, I studiously avoided shared spaces: the big table where patients congregated to watch the boxy dolly-mounted TV; and later, in the next ward I'd be admitted to, the TV and activity rooms where patients buzzed or lolled or sat. Introverted at my best, I spent my institutionalized time impotently attempting to construct personal spaces. Of course there is no me-space in a hospital, certainly not if you've been certified as posing a danger to yourself. No corner behind curtained dividers or unlatchable doors to effectively mark one's own. As my eyes improved, I resorted to my childhood proclivity for disappearing into books, pulling my consciousness through that escape hatch and shutting it behind me.

I was hardly a sociable patient, hardly the one to get psych-evaluation bonus points for successful interpersonal interactions.

Hardly the insatiably curious inveterate reporter I'd fancied myself before entering that building.

I encountered insomnia without end, twisting on squeaky hospital linen, shallow sleep interrupted by what I thought was the rolling sound of gurneys thundering through hallways but turned out to be the trundling pneumatic whoosh of specimens, samples, medication sent from one ward to another through a tube system within the walls. When I could sleep I'd dream I was trapped and tied down in a maze-like Mengele hospital where maniacs conducted sadistic experiments. It was almost a relief to be roused in the morning by nurses bearing thermometers and blood-pressure cuffs. Almost, but for the perma-fatigue that lodged itself in my joints and behind my eyes.

I grew to love the hospital's intercom announcements. Code Blue for cardiac arrest; Code White for a violent patient; Code Yellow for a missing person, an elopee, as they're called, a runaway for whom I'd silently cheer. *Go, sixty-eight-year-old Caucasian man with short brown hair last seen wearing hospital pants and a brown wool cardigan and no shoes! Run!*

Days were divided between Visiting Hours and Everything Else. My baby sister flew in, too beautiful and young and on the cusp of life to have to worry about this shit barely a month after I'd schlepped a printer uphill to her McGill University residence in Montreal. The five of us—my parents, brother, sister and I—went outside the hospital for meals and pretended everything was fine. We went for a late brunch on Queen Street West and sat in a corner table by the window and all ordered variations on the same huevos rancheros and my dad bought a stranger's black-and-white photos. Their outward resilience and our collective ability to laugh at the most horrible things helped me get through without choking on my own guilt.

These escorted outings were not carefree ones for my parents. "We were both happy to be there for you . . . but at the same time scared shitless," my dad said, years later. "You once went into the bathroom at a Queen Street restaurant where we were out for dinner and suddenly we were terrified that maybe you took a knife to the bathroom and were going to try to kill yourself again while on an escorted leave from hospital."

(I was oblivious to this. I just went to the bathroom.)

And my friends. I'd done nothing to deserve such stalwarts. Brendan brought me fancy overpriced sandwiches on the first day I was allowed a chaperoned out-of-ward excursion. I stood facing south on a bench in a green-space-cum-smoking-area near one of the hospital's entrances, fingertips upstretched to touch a vine-laced wooden trellis as I blinked like a mole rat in the honeyed evening light. I'd never had a brisket sandwich before and it remains the most delicious bread-based thing I've ever consumed. I hoarded half of it for later only to have it confiscated by well-meaning nurses who seemed to interpret my sentimentality in a more pathological way.

Omar, my closest friend and the most masochistic individual I know, came to hospital every goddamn day, even after I was moved upstairs to the ward for serious crazies. Every day! He signed me out and took me wandering through hospital hallways as I hyena-laughed uncontrollably, so stupid-glad to be with someone I loved who wasn't running away despite all available evidence and common sense and instinctive self-preservation advising the contrary. (The only evening he missed was the day Steve Jobs died, because he had to write about it.[5] Wesley came and braved the upstairs psych ward in his stead.) And as long as I returned from these brief respites to sign back in before my time was up, everything was okay. Pushing it once, trying to fit in two sign-outs too close together, aroused enough suspicion to temporarily cost me chaperoned sign-out privileges. I was left sulky and prowling for thirty hours, starved for fresh air.

Most of my psych-ward time was deadly cabin fever: marathon pacing, ear-splitting earbud music, books that were never escapist enough to hold my splintered attention for long. So despite attempts to retreat within myself, I got to know my fellow patients.

A Hispanic woman had family come visit en masse. They trooped in armed with pastries and tamales, filling the common area with chatter and warmth. She was one of the few inpatients who got many visitors. Watching the way she swelled with love when they were near, the way she wept later, alone and deflated, made it seem imperative that everything in her world turn out okay.

In the curtained bed space next to mine was an elderly woman, grey hair in a long braid slung over her shoulder. Her sling-clad arm was lined lengthwise with a thick spiderweb of angry black stitches I could not stop staring at. I'd imagine the scene at her home as she bled—did she call 911 herself? Had she changed her mind, was the sight of her own blood too much to bear? I knew she lived alone because I overheard a social worker talk to her at one point about learning to prepare her meals with one arm. She approached me one morning in the liminal space between our cubbyholes and asked me to adjust her sling and I tried to hide my fixation on her arm as I slipped the fabric into a slightly less uncomfortable space bracketing elbow and shoulder. (Following a knee surgery years later, I found the same sutures, a pair of baleful black knots, in my own skin while replacing one set of waterproof Band-Aids with another. Was astonished at the degree to which they froze me, took me back to that forlorn wrinkled old lady with the long grey hair and the thick spidery stitches crawling up her forearm. Did she have to go back to hospital to get them removed, as I did mine? Did she make the appointment? Follow-ups are a bitch at the best of times; surely far worse when it's to untie the sutures undoing your effort to die.)

At night her moans of discomfort roused me from whatever light doze I could manage, till I prayed for one or both of us to just shut up and die. In the morning, remorse at my murderous callousness prompted me to slip her, at her request, the packets of salt from my meal tray—she got none, for health reasons. Was I undermining her long-term wellness? Maybe. But when you're old and alone and in pain and stuck in hospital after trying to slit your wrist, surely there are more important things to worry about than sodium intake.

A nurse-chaperoned trip down to the hospital's belly for a brain scan felt like a vacation. I spent interminable minutes in a luminescent white *Space Odyssey* cocoon whose broad vocabulary of echoing blurps and bloops mimicked the sound effects of a retro sci-fi film. I learned the less-than-uplifting result of this diversion days later. An otherworldly neurologist—wide blue eyes growing wider, syncopated Scandinavian-accented voice slowing as she spoke—walked me through a series of white blobs I was told depicted my brain.

A dangly blob at the centre of the bird's-eye image she introduced to me as my putamen, located near the bottom of the brain itself. It was swollen thanks to the antifreeze I'd swallowed. I learned through later googling that, once in your system, the methanol in antifreeze metabolizes into formic acid, which can prevent your cells from grabbing and using the oxygen they need, ultimately killing you within about thirty-six hours.[6] Your optic nerve and basal ganglia are among the first bodily bits badly damaged in this process—either directly poisoned by formic acid or suffocated by lack of oxygen. Depending how badly damaged they are, you could be blind or shaky and off-balance for the rest of your life. I did not know this when I gulped that blue liquid. My pre-attempt googling fixated only on the prospect of death, not debilitation. I'd gone for what seemed both efficacious and accessible, with little thought for side effects. Smart!

I was unreasonably lucky, the neurologist told me, in a tone that suggested I should not tempt fate again: the damage to my basal ganglia was probably temporary, she advised. (She also advised me to avoid booze for the next several months. *What, you mean other than methyl alcohol?*) That swollen dangly blob, my putamen, explained my greater-than-usual klutziness; a damaged optic nerve could explain the watery stinging in my eyes every time I tried to focus. My swollen putamen also sabotaged my hands when I needed them most. For weeks I wrote and typed with agonizing, disorienting slowness, cramped fingers and crabbed letters not my own.

That panicky self-alienation dissipated after a couple of months, and by January follow-up brain scans found my putamen had recovered as much as it ever will. I discovered soon after that I could no longer pull off high heels when I toppled over like a drunken pygmy giraffe while walking fifty metres to a wedding venue. Red-faced and mortified I picked myself up, cradling my miraculously unshattered camera and avoiding eye contact, slunk back to the vehicle I'd carpooled in to retrieve a pair of flat sandals. (For the record, I temporarily relearned how to walk in heels for my baby brother's 2017 wedding and remain absurdly proud of myself for not sprawling across the aisle or crushing small children on the dance floor.) Some necrotic-looking scar tissue remains, nerve fibres stripped of their white myelin insulation. Insidious symptoms persist: I still get freaky limb microtremors, jackhammer legs, shaky hands that shake more thanks to certain psychotropic medications I've taken on and off for the past several years. Three-and-a-half years later, back in hospital following—SPOILER ALERT—another suicide attempt, a bemused doctor approached my ICU bed, scans in hand, wondering how a woman in her late twenties had the brain of a stroke victim. That's apparently what medical images of my brain look like to people who aren't expecting to encounter methanol's neurological souvenirs.

Back in the psych ward, I was acutely aware of my involuntary status and irrationally resentful of anyone there with me who was effectively free to go at any time. A young bearded man who'd voluntarily checked himself in to the short-term psych ward spent extensive amounts of time on the hospital phone talking about how he'd *just needed some time to decompress, you know?* He held forth at length on the quality and quantity of food he consumed and its variegated effects on his digestive system. It's vital for voluntary admission to be available to people in crisis—it's infinitely better than the alternative, of resources being unavailable or only available on an involuntary basis. But goddamn, I was so jealous.

Form 3 or no, I was sure if I just acted normal enough they would let me go. I tried to be courteous, lucid and calm but not suspiciously upbeat. I didn't weep or scream at my own frustration or impotence or exhaustion or insomnia or self-loathing. I met, as required, multiple times a day with nurses and social workers. And my I'm-totally-fine, suicide-was-a-one-time-aberration ploy almost worked: I was almost set free by the first psychiatrist I saw within a week of my admission without so much as a follow-up appointment.

I admit we got off on the wrong foot with that first psychiatrist. This could be because my family and I misjudged her appetite for jokes. The six of us—me, parents, siblings, psychiatrist—had a painful group session involving questions about not just me but family practices and dynamics. (I learned later on that my parents, as family members grasping for information and a meaningful sense of participation in their loved one's care, found this group session more useful than I did.) When substance use came up I recall my dad saying something along the lines of, "Do we drink? Oh, yeah. Allllll the time." And then we all chuckled while the psychiatrist sat stony-faced and made notes that, I later learned, branded us all alcoholics. Let me be clear: my family drinks regularly, especially when together. But none of us drink destructively. We don't get antsy-distressed when we go without booze. Clearly this is something I should have paused our psych-session wisecracking to clarify before the woman pathologized us all.

Anyway.

My discharge was scheduled, it shone like a beacon, with nothing more for me to deal with than a list of phone numbers of private pricey psychotherapists and the Centre for Addiction and Mental Health, whose wait list for a publicly covered post-suicide psychiatric consultation stretched past six weeks. I dutifully made these calls from behind my blue curtain, voice comically lowered as I shamefully booked appointments with several psychotherapists I hoped my employer would pay for even as I recoiled from the idea of couch-bound confessions, knowing I'd distance myself from everything to do with this horrid experience as soon as possible.

Incidentally, discharging inpatients who have mental disorders requiring ongoing treatment with a series of phone numbers and a pat on the head is not considered best practice: it's a great way to ensure people fall through the cracks and (if they're lucky) wind up back in hospital in worse shape than before. St Joe's, the hospital where I stayed, now has a mental health outpatient clinic that focuses in part on catching people at risk of death or deterioration as they head back into the community. Hooking people up with ongoing care, making the transition as seamless as possible, makes for better outcomes—and, hopefully, fewer fatally shitty ones. Yet somehow ensuring smooth psych transitions remains the exception, not the rule. It's a hospital-dependent crapshoot.

My parents—who'd been driven nuts by the sense of enforced helplessness and ignorance they had to live with as family members of mental patients who by law retain their right to privacy—thought setting me free less than a week after a suicide attempt was a bad idea. We had a bruising shouting match, pacing back and forth in sinking damp sand by Lake Ontario, near the path we walked during my all-too-brief afternoon chaperoned psych-ward reprieves, arguing over whether I should live with them in Vancouver on my release. I wanted to go home to my apartment. But I admit my argument was less than compelling:

"I'm fine!"

"That's what you said before you tried to kill yourself."

"But now I really am fine!"

My parents won that argument, albeit not in the way they—or I—expected.

3

Psych-Ward Sojourn

Unbeknownst to me, as I paced by my bed and prepared for life outside the windowless ward, my parents had pushed for a second opinion, my dad writing desperate, pleading emails at three o'clock in the morning. And they got one.

The second psychiatrist was smart and sardonic and treated me like someone capable of communicating in multisyllabic sentences. He also had a far better bullshit-detector. He did not buy my argument that this whole suicide thing was an anomalous one-off, a mental misunderstanding, never to recur. He decided I had major depression. And that I was fucked-up enough to merit more time locked up lest I try to off myself again.

So much for my "suicide, shmuicide" master plan. The people charged with keeping me alive were not so easily convinced.

Years later I still resent his decision to keep me locked up, even though his intervention also earned me invaluable outpatient care and years of life-ameliorating, arguably lifesaving treatment. He also got me started on meds, the beginning of a years-long pill-popping parade, on which more later. This was the doctor I would see as an outpatient, who would help me stay alive in the most basic way for years. But I still don't think I needed more time in a mental institution—I think I could have started one-on-one outpatient pharmaco- and psychotherapy sooner and skipped the extra time in the ward and gotten more benefit from it without risking another self-administered death. He still contends that keeping me in a psych ward was the right move because I was at a high risk of attempting suicide after what he concluded was a serious and premeditated attempt—apartments don't get to that state in a day, and telling him gulping antifreeze was a freak impulsive act "would have been a whole lot easier to argue if you drove a car," he said. My attempt at a model-patient persona was not how people who attempted suicide on impulse tend to act. Letting me go at that point "would have been a premature discharge." And premature discharges in all contexts are of course to be avoided.

But at the time I just about broke down. Agape as my discharge—which was scheduled, which I'd prepped for—was delayed, I struggled to process the prospect of more time without freedom of movement, more sleepless hospital nights. I squandered precious visiting hours pacing the three-step space along my bed. In hindsight I can see it seems an overreaction but at the time I was distraught, unable to bear the company of loved ones who could come and go as they chose.

Within hours of my getting the unwelcome news, a well-meaning patient advocate whose business card I promptly lost took me aside and explained I could appeal, if I wanted, to the Consent and Capacity Board. That board, he explained, made up of psychiatrists, lawyers and laypersons, is where you go when there's a disagreement over how crazy you are or who should get to decide on treatment if a patient herself can't. I later found its caseload more than doubled in the decade ending in 2016–17:[1] the biggest portion of its applications (46 percent in 2016–17) dealing with patients' involuntary status. The onus is on the attending doctor, the one who put you on the Form, to prove you should be there. I spent a day considering trying to challenge my commitment. By this time I'd been in hospital just over a week, but I still hoped somehow good behaviour would earn me a clean bill of health and quicker return to the newsroom. (Also, by then I'd lost that guy's card.)

So I got myself set to move to the long-term psych ward upstairs.

I packed the too many belongings I'd accumulated—books and clothes, but also the rosemary plant from my mother, the stuffed monster and fuzzy slippers from friends—into too few plastic bags. With a nurse at my side I trekked upstairs, looking every bit a dishevelled bag lady—a parody of a poor soul who belongs somewhere closed off and sedated.

THE SEVENTH-FLOOR PSYCH WARD—7M, it's called—was a converted brick-gabled nunnery at the top of the hospital. And I will give it this: it had a lovely view, catching morning sun and evening sun and the glinting, traffic-rimmed Lake Ontario to the south. I got a chance to admire this view for the first time as I fidgeted in the TV alcove while my possessions were taken away and protractedly combed through. I stood by a window near the bland square side table and the unstainable blue-green L-shaped couch, avoiding eye contact with the patients watching TV beside me or reading, sitting and staring, or playing games in the larger adjoining activity room, used breakfast trays stacked in a tall wheeled cart in the corner. They let me keep my shoelaces and earbuds but confiscated spare hair elastics and charger cords, along with the nail polish my younger sister had given me and the jar of apple butter from my mother—part of her ongoing attempt to make my psych-ward sojourn as homey as possible. Unquenchable nesting instinct! Were I on death row or locked in solitary I'm certain she'd bring me a potted plant, yoga mat, prints for the walls or a beach-glass mobile to hang from the ceiling.

The nurse who led me to my latchless, off-white room advised me to keep all my possessions locked for safekeeping in the vertical cupboard to which the nurses kept the key.

"Oh, are many things stolen here?"

"Oh, yes."

The sureness of her response, that implied inevitability of theft, sparked an immediate suspicion of my fellow inmates. Unwarranted: the only thing anyone ever stole from my room was some fruit.

My quarters resembled, really, a spartan university dorm room: bed, desk, chair, cupboard/wardrobe. On the walls were scrawled disappointingly uncreative rants, much of it written in the same ball-point pen, mostly combinations of homages to and warnings against Satan. I spent too many time-killing hours engaged in morbid hand-writing analysis, comparing the sole pencilled set of rantings to the satanic ballpoint pen. Same person, different implement? Different person, same crazed uncreativity? The myth of the mad creative genius makes for good narratives but in my experience it's a myth. I know brilliant people who have mental illness but the latter is a bug, not a feature. Psychic torment punches you in the face and crowbars you in the knees; it doesn't make you Mensa magic. Maybe some lucky nutbars have the productive-creative-brilliant brand of crazy. But the only reason it seems an inordinate number of artsy genius types are crazy is because you never hear from us normal crazy people. All those tortured brainiacs are far outnumbered by poor fuckers who're just tortured. Mental illness made me incurious, inert. I retreated into myself. I struggled to write. I could not take notes, despite my grandmother's advice. Even outside hospital, in the months before my first suicide attempt and the years afterward, the deepen-ing of suicidal despair drowned out any creativity or curiosity I thought I had even as I struggled to keep pitching, keep chasing, keep filing. My handwriting's never been legible but my swollen putamen made my hand muscles seize up and rebel. To see words I'd written sprawl unrecognizable like pulverized mosquitos across a page was terrifying and disorienting and made me even more reluctant to record anything.

The bed was pushed lengthwise against the east-facing window whose lower half, for some reason, was tinted. I caused one poor nurse minor panic when I stood on the bed for a better view of the traffic wormtrails seven storeys below, leaving only part of my torso (The strangulation-by-hanging part, right?) visible from the hallway through the small window in my door. But there were precious few ligature opportunities to be had in that convent enclave. Not that I was actively looking, but it was hard not to think about, a niggling errand you'd rather ignore but that keeps presenting itself, in the same way I joked with Omar about testing the tensile strength of the headphones they let me keep. I really was joking but also wondered—could I use them?

None of the doors locked and they didn't latch shut properly either—not mine, not the washroom's, not the shower room's where the wooden urine-scented bench lent a deceptively sauna-y air of class, as though it belonged in the mountain chateau of a senile, eccentric old man. Showers were a daily failed attempt to put my change of clothes somewhere they wouldn't get soaked; I wasn't about to trudge through that hall wearing nothing but a hospital-issued towel.

To enter the ward from the seventh-floor elevator you needed to be beeped in by whomever was (wo)manning a nurses' station beyond the heavy locking glass doors with their "WATCH FOR ELOPEES" sign. No one eloped, or tried to, while I was in that ward. I kept wishing someone would.

The tiled whitish hallway leading to the patient rooms smelled eternally of piss thanks to an incontinent, bedridden, birdlike old lady across from the nurses' station. The space was nonetheless perpetually teeming with patients milling about or waiting to use the phone or seeking a nurse's attention. We were each assigned a nurse in the morning, based on who was working that day, names written in blue on a whiteboard like awkward workplace team-building assignments. Each nurse had a handful of inpatient charges and you were supposed to address any concerns/complaints/requests to your designated nurse of the day. Attempting to talk to anyone else elicited a terse "I am not your nurse!" and a quickly receding back. I know you don't want a bedlam of patients shouting at random people in uniforms. But this felt damn infantilizing.

The doors to everyone's room were rarely open unless there were nurses inside checking vitals or administering meds or haranguing ambulatory patients out of bed. You'd think a psych ward would be the one place it's acceptable to stay in bed and wallow in your own misery. But no. Orderlies changed sheets and garbage and, if you caught them at the right time, your towel for a fresh one. One nurse showed me the rumbling industrial washer and dryer down the hall where they washed the linen and where I could do my own laundry. Never before or since has this seemed such a privilege.

There was a caged-off balcony facing south, toward the highway and the water, which was open to inmates for a few minutes a day if we could successfully prevail upon the nurses. I gazed at the Gardiner Expressway and longed to be stuck among the glittering lines of vehicles stretching east and west alongside the shining surface of Lake Ontario. During one of these all-too-brief moments of fresh air I struck up a conversation with the woman in charge of the hospital's psych wards, who'd come to the seventh floor for a brief visit. We talked about her responsibilities at the hospital, about her cat and her Thanksgiving plans. The exchange ended abruptly when the nurses ushered everyone back inside and I was reminded I was not an independent person, not a curious reporter, but a crazy person on a Form who could not be trusted on her own.

One exception to my studious avoidance of fellow inmates— a foray into the long-term psych ward's common room to play Scrabble—ended abortively when my opponent's word choices took a turn for the rapey. I freaked and retreated to my unlockable room. (I should add, in fairness, I was never given any concrete reason to fear for my safety while an inpatient. Most of the other psych-ward denizens were much more sociable and solicitous than I was. But this was an unnerving moment in an unnerving setting, so. On the bright side, I didn't get a chance to lose: I suck at Scrabble.)

The ward psychiatrist would call each of us in for periodic chats in a cramped bright space between the elevator and the common room. "How is your *mood*?" she'd ask each time, and I tried to sound just upbeat enough for my reply not to ring fake ("I saw the sunrise this morning! It was beautiful!").

I don't know what kind of treatment most of my fellow inmates were getting. Apart from those psychiatric chats there were mandatory life-skills activities like the nutritional bingo delivered by an overly perky, heavily pregnant young woman whose cheery patience was wasted on most of us. I saw a couple of patients frighteningly woozy on meds, but that was it. More than anything else the place felt like a holding pen—a drunk tank for crazy. You could be there for weeks or months but it wasn't a place you were meant to live.

I spent most of the vast empty stretches between visiting hours reading in my room or reading on the floor, tucked into a semi-sunny corner beside the glass balcony door, a sad-eyed hound hoping someone will notice her and let her out (it was here I fell in love with Esi Edugyan's fiction). The lack of agency was the worst, of course. That, and the lack of privacy. That, and the lack of fresh air that almost drove me to start smoking so at least I could steal a bit of extra time outdoors for nurse-chaperoned nicotine outings. (I've since been informed those no longer exist. Too many elopees.)

Shortly after my move to 7M a senior editor from the paper came to visit. Old-school, in charge of something amorphous like the newspaper's editorial standards, stern-seeming unless you knew her. She came in the late afternoon or early evening and I got my parents to sign me out of the nuthouse so I could meet her in the cramped ground-floor hospital coffee shop instead of the psych ward's septic-antiseptic common room.

I was petrified. I'm sure it showed. But god, that visit meant so much it beggars verbalizing. She came and brought chocolate and newsroom gossip and we sipped coffee and talked about news and politics and who'd had a baby, who was out of his depth in a new job. And I remember palpably trembling, from meds or anxiety or both, and praying she didn't notice and that I didn't seem too crazy (*Do I seem crazy now? How about now? Howaboutnow?*). If I did she was gracious enough not to let on. At one point I tried to clumsily apologize without really specifying what for: neither of us had uttered the word "suicide" and I certainly wouldn't be the one to haul it into a conversation teetering perilously on the cordially sane. She brushed it off: "Everyone's allowed a couple of screw-ups." "This is a pretty big screw-up." She laughed. We talked about my return to work as though it were a real, imminent thing, not a delusional fantasy. I said the doctors thought being posted to a foreign bureau would be therapeutic. She laughed. I pretended that what I interpreted as the laughability of that ambition wasn't breaking my heart. I don't know what it took for her to come and visit me in hospital. But I experienced it as a gift, a superhuman act of kindness. It made me feel like a real person with a vocation and aspirations to return to. I grasped at that feeling in the days and weeks afterward, a bright thread in a dark labyrinth.

DEMOCRACY IS THE BEST. I woke on Ontario election day with devastation down my insides: I was supposed to be covering this story, not watching it sidelong from a psych ward. But there was a silver lining, under the circumstances: freedom. Canadian inpatients, like prison inmates, retain their right to vote even while they've temporarily lost their right to freedom of movement. I unearthed my voter information card, requisite identification and proof of address; negotiated an extended leave—two consecutive hours!—from the psych ward and walked to my polling station to cast a vote. Most of my ward didn't know an election was ongoing (notable exception: the wonderful lady who bellowed, "Who won the election?" from her room the following morning), or knew they could vote, or where they could vote, assuming they had a driver's licence, health card, mail addressed to their permanent residence handy. Everyone who'd been committed would have needed chaperones. I had the good fortune of being accompanied by my parents, who took their guardianship role verrrry seriously. They all but held my hand as we crossed the street.

I've always loved polling stations and ballot-casting. But the normalcy, the heady sense of democracy in action is so much sweeter when there's no one asking you if you're planning to end your life, if you've taken your meds, if you're allowed to be out. To the genial

Elections Ontario workers I was just one more smiley voter, with a slight tremor you'd only notice if you looked really closely.

On our way back, aglow with the glory of participatory democracy and ready to leap to the barricades, we stopped at a No Frills to pick up toiletries. Conditioner was on sale (a big deal when you have long curly Wookiee hair) and I weighed the family-size bottles in my hands, wondering whether to buy a second. "Do it!" my mom urged. "You're going to be alive a long time!" At that moment, in my mind, that cheery prognosis became a threat, a trap, a heavy door clanging shut. I wanted to scream and run away, evade my own powerlessness. I grabbed my conditioner and headed to the checkout.

Back on the ward, my best friend among the seventh-floor patients, a jokey, grizzled man who wore loose drawstring pyjama pants and little else, was kind enough to change the channel on the wall-mounted TV I couldn't reach from hockey to the election coverage. He watched the results trickle in with me, making genial, racist remarks about the ethnic-sounding names of various candidates. He bragged about his near-death heroin overdoses, his karate-practising grandchildren, the pot he'd somehow managed to smuggle onto the ward.

Even an anti-social glued-to-her-book recluse like me needed an ally for the twelve waking hours every day without visitors. Grizzly Dude and I would bellow at each other down the off-beige hall, "What, are you *crazy*?!" and guffaw as though we were world-class comedians and not sad-sack psych-ward inmates. We tried and failed to muffle our laughter at the bizarre weekly discussion circles, meant as an opportunity for inmates to air living-condition grievances but really more like a parody of Ken Kesey's *One Flew Over the Cuckoo's Nest*. When I didn't materialize to grab my breakfast tray (which was every morning: the food was consistently, comically awful; a mushy bland caricature of hospital grub) he sometimes brought it to my room.

And then suddenly it was Thanksgiving, and we each got a pass to escape the ward over the long weekend—he to stay with his mom and attend her celebratory dinner, me to stay with my parents in the place they were renting for the duration of my little meltdown. It was a weird weekend. I still had to be chaperoned everywhere by a putatively responsible adult. My dad jogged along when I went for a run in the morning; a coterie of friends picked me up and drove me to a hiking spot outside the city and I stood in the parking lot with my face upturned to the sun like I was attempting photosynthesis. I had coffee with a co-worker who told me we couldn't be friends anymore, not close friends, because it hurt too much. (Can't say I blame her but that just about broke me.) I tagged along with Omar to a painfully awkward corporate PR party—"Do you want to come with me to this?" "Uh, this is Anna. Did you mean to call somebody else?"— where bands squawked under circling coloured disco lights in a fire-hazardous converted warehouse as I, newly teetotalling, nabbed miniature hamburgers off serving trays. I had less agency over my movements than at any time since I was eight years old, and felt it. But the people I loved who upended commitments and turned their lives inside-out for me made those days bearable.

"We all felt if we could just show you how much we love you, how much we need you in our lives . . . it might not make you better, but maybe it would make you think twice about killing yourself," my dad told me years later.

The autumnal scenes from that weekend seem made for an idyllic montage in a cheesy movie. Misleadingly: outpatient downtime is a great opportunity to ruminate over your own monstrousness and mistakes and the hurt you've caused people you claim to love. I remember, vividly, lying on my side awake in bed, thinking for the first time post-antifreeze how best to kill myself, the need pressing like weight on a bladder. It was back.

My poor gorgeous siblings had decamped to school so it was a muted Thanksgiving dinner. My parents took the opportunity to ask me why I hadn't left a note.

What do you say to that? I said it seemed presumptuous to try to explain something I could sense would be inexplicable to the explanation's audience no matter what I said to try to justify causing this kind of hurt, knowing full well the hurt it would cause. I didn't say that note-leaving was not top of mind for me at that moment. But it has been since then. It occupies my thoughts in the days and hours when ending my life seems most urgently imperative. Who needs a note? What do I say? Should I leave them in envelopes at home? Mail them? What if I mail a note and then change my mind or screw up my death? How gross would that be? I've asked my more morbid-minded friends if they'd rather I left them a note but no one's been shameless enough to say. Does it make it better or worse, having a note from someone whose suicide has left you grieving? (I'm genuinely curious. Answer in the comment section below!)

We stopped on our way back to hospital to pick up a sack of bulk candy I'd promised Grizzly Dude. He was heartbreakingly pleased.

THE LONG-TERM PSYCH-WARD residents were several levels crazier than the short-term ward's patients. They also seemed to interact and pal around more, perhaps because they were there long enough to form friendships; perhaps because lunacy lowers social inhibitions (when it doesn't socially incapacitate you, as it did me). One young man with schizophrenia paced the halls wild-eyed, swearing under his breath for hours a day. He discomfited me at first but was harmless, although he's my primary suspect in the theft of a bag of Honeycrisp apples from my room, going solely on the hearsay of my grizzly patient friend. Most were comparatively subdued, moving between levels of lucidity. Most were men, most older than me. One of the only exceptions was a tiny young woman with close-cropped dark hair and a body of sharp angles, who had an eating disorder and a strained relationship with her family.

One loud, gangly man who stood in the common area declaring his schizophrenia ("I am schizophrenic, and so am I!") was clearly a regular. (I should maybe note that people with schizophrenia don't generally have multiple personalities.) He recalled previous incarnations of the ward's amenities—apparently the TV had improved; the pillows had not—when he served as jumpy secretary during weekly patient meetings. He told everyone in detail about his fungally infected foot, which needed its own special sandal. He stopped me and a visiting friend one evening to loudly proclaim his views on gay people (strongly disliked) and then Toronto mayor Rob Ford (strongly liked, although he seemed to think Ford was premier). He had a habit of staring at your chest and making grandiose rambling compliments, then elucidating his love for his wife—same script each time. He called his teenage son sometimes from the wall-mounted phone outside the nurses' station. Asked him to visit, bring him foot cream and other necessities. If the boy dropped by I didn't see him.

I don't envy anyone whose job it was to care for us in the long-term ward, babysitting a floor of complex, erratic, unwell individuals, many of whom would be better off elsewhere. There aren't enough intermediate- or long-term facilities for people who can't care for themselves but don't need to be hospitalized (more on that later). And my west-end Toronto hospital abuts Parkdale, a gentrifying neighbourhood of new immigrants, rising rents, trending restaurants, scuzzy apartment buildings, huge old subdivided houses and one of the highest concentrations of people battling addiction and crippling mental illness in the country—the second-highest rate of psychiatric hospital visits in the fourth-largest city on the continent.[2]

A few months before my suicide attempt, in the spring of 2011, Parkdale was terrorized by someone (or several people) attacking mentally ill residents seemingly at random.[3] I'd been living in the neighbourhood more than a year by the time that happened, a few lanes of highway between me and the blue dish of lake, and loved the community. I never felt unsafe but knew parents of young kids who'd found used needles in playgrounds. As so often happens, when the area cleans up, its most vulnerable residents get pushed out. In recent years rooming houses have been sold, rebranded and subdivided into micro-bachelor apartments renting for $1,300 a month.[4] But this is still where the services are—the community health centres, the legal clinic, employment and language and other social services—and this is where people grew up and found community so, as in any big city, they stick around to the extent they can, to the extent there's somewhere affordable and accessible to live or sleep or crash.

An inordinate proportion of my hospital's psychiatric inpatients were (are) homeless; many brought there by police, who I've been told go out of their way to drop people off at this crisis unit rather than others because of its rapid processing times. The hospital gets more of these police drop-offs than any other facility in the city, despite having far fewer psychiatric beds than other places, such as the prominent Centre for Addiction and Mental Health.[5] I once talked to a recovering lifelong alcoholic in Parkdale who, when he was going through a particularly bad withdrawal, which happened a fair bit, would try to get paramedics to take him to St. Joe's rather than elsewhere because he knew he'd be treated compassionately. I still see people in the neighbourhood—walking down the street, waiting for a streetcar, grabbing a coffee or a sandwich—I recognize from the outpatient mental health clinic where I, too, am now a regular. And some people keep checking themselves back in. They've nowhere else to go. This is the home address they put on whatever forms they're required to fill out because it's the closest place they have. Many of the long-term ward's inhabitants cycle through endlessly—too needy to live alone, not needy enough to need hospitalization, no one to advocate on their behalf for supportive housing and nowhere near enough social housing to go around. There are a hundred thousand people on that waiting list in Toronto alone.[6] Housing, especially supportive housing—proven umpteen times to improve health care, corrections, social outcomes[7]—is still something we're terrible at providing for those who need it most.

Surely, few groups of patients are as unpleasant by definition as those whose disease targets their brains. If it's weird waking to find yourself in a different stranger's care each morning, it can't be much more pleasant to be charged with caring for a cycle of erratic nutbars with sub-optimal hygiene practices. One friendly night nurse told me he'd come to Canada to work in literature after winning awards for his writing and translating in China. Turns out it's easier to get a gig as a nurse than as a Chinese–English translator though, so he went back to school and swapped planned translations of Atwood, Richler, Munro for shifts with pissy psych inpatients. I wish I'd asked what he was reading. A Filipino Canadian nurse I tried unsuccessfully to cajole into casting a ballot was worried her two kids would emerge from post-secondary with degrees and no jobs.

I forgot everyone's name.

AT THE END of my two-week Form 3, the "How is your mood?" ward psychiatrist decided I was free to go. I'm not sure whether this was motivated more by my progress or their need for beds. I didn't feel better, particularly; suicide didn't seem like an immediate option but nothing seemed like much of an immediate option. I hadn't processed the prospect of putting my life back together. But I didn't care. The feeling of being No Longer Certifiable was fantastic. My parents were coming to pick me up. They would help me find a new apartment and then decamp across the country to Vancouver. "The hardest thing," my mom later told me, "was leaving you [in Toronto] by yourself. You were very independent and strong . . . but I also wanted to look after you and keep you safe. But I couldn't. . . .

"We came to realize how helpless we were, and that was—apart from the fact of knowing that we could lose you at any time—that was the hardest thing to deal with. . . . [Being] powerless in a role where we felt it's our responsibility to help you and keep you safe."

Reading books about depression helped her feel informed, but also terrified.

"You never want to accept the fact that your kid could kill herself." Long pause. "So I try to be positive. I don't dwell on that too much."

"I HOPE I NEVER see you again," my nurse of the day said. It was sunny. I got my bike back. Everything was going to be okay.

4

What, Me Depressed?

You'll want to know when and you'll want to know why.

When everyday pissiness gave way to ineluctable despair.

Why I tried, repeatedly, to fix it by killing myself.

The answer is I don't know. Not to any half-satisfactory degree. Certainly not the second question. Not even the first, really. As much as I wind my mind back in time I'm unable to locate the start of a downward spiral. And every well-meaning therapeutic discussion I've had attempting to dredge childhood trauma proves futile and guilt-inducing. I've never been subject to anything awful enough to warrant this mind-swallowing badness. I have a supportive, loving family, had a happy childhood. I'm a very fortunate person. Only problem is, I hate myself and want to die.

Mental illness, strictly speaking, doesn't run in my family. Are there people in my family a psychiatrist might diagnose with something like an anxiety disorder, if they got the opportunity? Probably.

And nothing prompts disclosures like one's own very public, very ugly mental breakdown: One relative admitted to me shortly after my first suicide attempt her own bedridden-paralysis feeling; another told me about her anxiety, which she successfully kept at bay with tiny doses of a common antidepressant I wish worked that magic on me; another took antidepressants for years, although by now he's taking such a wild combination of meds no one, his physicians included, has any idea what most of them do or how they work together.

But no one in my family has tried to kill herself; no one's had a psychotic break. No one's been hospitalized for psychiatric reasons. I'd call us neurotic in the casual, layperson sense but I can't point to any pathological history that could give clues to my medical misery.

I don't know where you'd mark my disorder's germination: When I began to have trouble waking up? (Maybe two years before my first suicide attempt?) When I began to dread going in to work, the thing that gave—gives—my life purpose? (Maybe eighteen months before?) When the smothering sense of failure prompted sporadic suicidal fantasies? (A year?) When those fantasies became insistent, persistent, inescapable?

My mother goes much earlier, to my teenage years. "I don't think it just came out of the blue," she said some seven years after that first attempt. She recalls a teen who withdrew and stopped eating, just about, for years. Who wore a back brace for scoliosis that became painfully uncomfortable and made adolescent awkwardness excruciating. "So even though we weren't maybe aware that what we were dealing with was depression, I think there were indicators. It seemed to me that you were dissatisfied with yourself from the time you were a teenager."

I've never liked myself much, as a person, and what my psychiatrist calls my "negative cognitive bias" probably stretches back to childhood. But when did I lose my capacity for hope?

I know that the attempt, when it came, felt long overdue—an inevitable, necessary step I couldn't keep putting off.

But I wouldn't have called myself depressed. Not when I decided I had to die and felt that conviction grow in intensity over the course of a year; not when my failed attempt left me in a psych ward answering awkward questions about my state of mind. The subsuming despondence, the inescapable hopelessness and worthlessness, were matters of fact: I existed without worth or hope.

Months before that first suicide attempt, presciently worried colleagues propelled into action by self-threatening emails had dragged me to the psych emerg and browbeaten me into calling my newspaper's employee assistance program. Which I did, and set up an appointment with a psychotherapist—for which I arrived, predictably, a half-hour late and which, predictably, I did not reschedule when the receptionist told me I'd arrived too late to see the therapist. I was relieved to have dropped the ball. Of course I couldn't get treatment. My despair was a pit dug by my own failures, not a remediable medical condition.

I couldn't believe my problem was extrinsic. I wanted to die because I was an idiot and could never improve, never move forward or do better—not because I was sick and therefore locked in a skewed perception of the world and myself within it.

It's not just me. Again and again, people I've spoken to bring up their sense of isolation, that theirs is a personal flaw unique to themselves, not something faced by others, certainly not something fixable. Debilitation—that inability to get out of bed, to interact with people—fuels self-revulsion. I loathed myself for the endless stasis, projects unrealized and opportunities ungrasped. I felt I was expending all my energy on the most basic level of functioning and had nothing to show for it—just years of going through the motions. And the worse I felt, the less motivated I was to pursue treatments that felt ineffectual.

So I resisted diagnosis. Even when a trained medical professional with decades of clinical psychiatric experience sat across from me informing me I had major depressive disorder, I resisted. "You have depression" did not strike me as a plausible explanation for what I was going through.

5

When Diagnosis Makes You Crazy

At first I resisted diagnosis because being diagnosed as mentally disordered meant more time spent hospitalized against my will. Sitting perched on the short-term psych ward's consult-room couch I was so close to freedom I could see it in the light sneaking through the hinges of the ward's weighted grey auto-locking door and I knew I had to be the most well-adjusted, healthy-seeming post-suicide girl you'd ever seen. Of course I rejected diagnosis: in addition to believing my problems were of my own making, I believed that diagnosis would keep me hospitalized indefinitely.

And I resisted because no one wants to be designated crazy and all that comes with it: that litany of off-putting, erratic, socially unacceptable behaviours; to be deemed dangerous, disposed toward violence and harm, to freakish unpredictability. I didn't want to be considered damaged, unhinged from reality. The patent ass-backwardness of those assumptions doesn't ease their stranglehold on a society that minimizes the medical toll of mental illness while maximizing its fear of those affected.

But maybe most of all I disdained my diagnosis because depression's a weak name for a serious disease. (I use "disease" and "illness" and "malady" as a layperson, more or less interchangeably in this book.)

You say "depression" and I think of Marvin the Paranoid Android. That endearing, hyper-intelligent robot from Douglas Adams' *The*

Hitchhiker's Guide to the Galaxy boasts the buzzkill tagline, "I think you ought to know I'm feeling very depressed." Marvin's a capable, dour, smart-aleck machine who solves foolish human problems even as he rolls his eyes at those humans' silly fallibility. He isn't a knot of despair consumed by worthlessness and failure. Beneath my external nope-I'm-totally-fine-please-discharge-me denial, I kept thinking, *That's it?* This emotional vacuum, this endless inescapable joyless negation of hope is just depression? Are you joking?

People profess depression all the time. Gloomy weather, inadequate investments in public transit, politically expedient xenophobia, the endangered status of a green-haired turtle that can breathe through its genitals'—they're all "depressing." It doesn't help that it's entirely possible to experience many of the symptoms of depression without being psychologically unwell: you can be anxious, you can doubt or reproach yourself, you can gain or lose weight, you can have trouble sleeping—and not have depression.

The official-sounding medical term, major depressive disorder, carries little extra gravitas, sounding more like the imaginings of a fanciful hypochondriac, not a genuine illness that does real harm. Surely, if what I had was a real disease and not simply justifiable despair at my own failure, it had to be something more serious.

One of psychiatry's most persistent bogeymen, dating to the mid-twentieth century and the basis of a still-burgeoning antipsychiatry movement, is the fear of turning normal human emotions into disorders.

But here's the thing: if the way I feel is just part of being human, for fuck's sake give me death. I cannot countenance the assertion that this hopeless chasm is simply an extreme on a spectrum of healthy emotion. It has no relation, however distant, to sadness. Sadness is a pain that reminds me I'm alive, that I'm an animal capable of emotion and a sense of loss. Despondence is the flat parched death of the soul. There's nothing there.

My dad remembers diagnosis differently. Remembers me telling him, while I was in that psych ward, that I'd been told I had depression.

"Hearing you acknowledge that you were sick was a big turning point, a really big moment. Because it wasn't a doctor telling us, it wasn't [your mother] or I making that lay conclusion. It was you, I guess, taking ownership of your own health and of your own state. So we weren't guardians of an unwilling individual anymore.

"By acknowledging you had an illness it was the first step you had to take to begin your process of recovery, I guess. . . . I saw the antifreeze. I saw the empty bottle of sleeping pills. I saw the apartment in disarray. I saw you literally fighting for your life as they tried to get the poisons out of your body. I saw you hot and sweaty and suffering in that ICU bed for a day. I knew you were sick. But I guess I was hoping that a diagnosis would lead to some kind of a cure. There was hope for recovery because we knew what was wrong."

It's never been that simple.

If existing definitions are flawed, and diagnostic methods hit and miss, the names we assign mood disorders often feel like a smokescreen masking costly ignorance: we group symptoms and call them an illness because we don't know how else to define the illness or address the symptoms.

This isn't rocket science: rocket scientists know how rockets work. The best psychiatrists in the world know astonishingly little about how the brain functions on a good day, let alone how it becomes diseased and how to treat it when it does. They don't know where depression comes from, or precisely how to map it in the brain, or why some interventions work, on some people, sometimes.

So where does that leave the diagnosed?

6

Killing Yourself Is Tougher
Than You'd Think

As I moped in the nunnery-cum–psych ward following my first blue antifreeze–flavoured attempt, I told myself and the psychiatrists deciding whether I was sane enough to be set free that there was no danger of my trying again. That, having failed so blatantly, with such unpleasant (but extraordinarily fortuitous, under the circumstances) after-effects, even similar feelings of despair wouldn't prompt me to attempt death again. That, effectively, I'd exhausted that option and was ready to move on to another, less lethal one.

I honestly believed this to be true. There's nothing like marinating in the guilt and self-disgust of one's botched suicide, wrapped in an ass-displaying blue hospital smock as earnest health workers monitor your blood pressure and probe your emotions, to convince you that you never want to try anything like that again.

But then you're out and all the awful comes rushing back.

No one tells you that after trying to kill yourself and failing miserably, you don't necessarily wake up in the ICU feeling awesome. No one tells you that, sometimes, you make it through two and a half weeks in two mental wards and back to the newsroom you love, only to be preoccupied with nothing so much as the wish you'd succeeded. Because everything that made you loathe yourself before is still there. Except now you're the crazy freak who can't even kill herself properly, who takes meds every morning that seem to do nothing, who's been away from work for a month and returns to pitch stories to someone who found her passed out and overdosed in her apartment. Chasing your vocation's a powerful protective factor. But being thrown back into it after an inpatient stay highlighted the agonizing delta between the person I perceived myself to be and the person I wanted to be.

I believe I wasn't at an elevated risk of suicide in the immediate aftermath of my first attempt. The weeks and months following, however, were another story.

FOR THE RECORD, I didn't really try to kill myself again for another year or so. I ducked down, powered through, tried to slough off the torpor that hijacked most days. Then, in the wake of another immobilized morning, steeped in shame at the electoral financing article I hadn't filed, I tried to smash my bedroom window with my desk chair. My chair is a lovely solid wooden thing. The windows in my apartment don't open—fruits of a compromise between the building's developer and the owners of a rubber plant next door who worried about the effect their fumes would have on north-facing residents. But I figured I could shatter that double-paned window and leap out to my death seventeen storeys below.

This did not work. Real-life windows are strong. I am not. Action movies lie. After a few futile swings barely left a scratch, I gave up and swallowed a month's worth of lithium, which I'd been prescribed at the time as an adjunct to antidepressants. Sat crouched by my bed, waiting for death and ignoring friends' frenzied phone calls wondering why I'd been incommunicado all day. Similarly ineffectual: fewer than fifteen minutes later my gastrointestinal tract's gag-reflex peristalsis betrayed me again. I was stuck sitting on my futon-couch, puke flecks studding my jeans, trying and failing to explain myself to my poor beloved friends who'd finally barged in.

I learned very quickly who was safe to confide in. Which friends would judge, flee, insist on calling my parents or the police. Which would listen, tell me they loved me, let me crash on their couch, without getting me in trouble. Maybe it's unfair—to sometimes need someone to confide in while also needing that person to take no drastic action in response to that confidence. But, again and again, that's where I found myself.

Then there were the asphyxiation attempts. I mutilated perfectly good plastic bags in my clumsy attempts to seal them airtight around my head with tape or elastic or knots only to realize I'd ripped holes in the motherfuckers. Following one such endeavour I bawled on a friend's shoulder in the middle of the night on a bench in a bright-lit twenty-four-hour supermarket, picking bits of scotch tape out of my hair to a piped-in generic pop soundtrack.

I was a toxicological ignoramus with an illogical aversion to outright googling "ways to kill yourself at home without a gun or any weight-bearing structure to facilitate strangulatory ligatures." So I'd do sidelong searches. "Toxic household chemicals." "Fatal X overdose," where X was whatever I was being prescribed at the time. I'd look up academic papers for lethal doses of whatever substances seemed easily obtainable and try to reverse-engineer blood concentration measurements to figure out how much of a given substance I'd need to ingest. I spent eternal minutes in the aisles of cavernous hardware stores, peering at warning labels and calculating how much I'd have to swallow, how quickly, how long it would take to work. Wondering if I looked as suspicious as I felt. I once bought a family-size pack of rat poison but couldn't bring myself to down the piles of pink and blue pellets sealed in clear plastic packets like heteronormative baby-shower loot bags. I tossed a fistful into a glass of water to soak, as though I'd feel better about ingesting them in soggy pablum form. They sat there bloating on the kitchen counter for a couple of days before I dumped them out, washed the glass obsessively, pretended it never happened.

I tried paint thinner. Don't try paint thinner. I managed to down barely a cup (okay, maybe a cup and a half) before the oily viscosity became too much.

I sat on my bed, looking out the window, trying to read Marjane Satrapi's graphic memoir *Persepolis* for more than an hour before I admitted defeat. Wept, went for a walk. It sounds horrible to say this but the conviction that one can't kill oneself despite wanting desperately to die is infinitely worse than the desire to die and the intention to follow through. Planning suicide at least gives you something to plan: once that's gone and the inclination remains, you have nothing.

It's from this abyss that I'd call a friend. Brendan, the first hapless mofo to answer the phone post–paint thinner, was covering a baseball game—could he call back? I wandered outside, bathed in evening light, palate coated with solvent. The fresh air reminded me I'd not eaten all day. Devoured whatever junk was in the fridge and the renewed gastric motility was enough to haul all that paint thinner back up. (There's a lot of puking in this book. I know. I apologize. But, honestly: poisoning's the leading method of suicide and suicide attempts among North American women. What were you expecting?)

Don't try paint thinner. Even after expelling everything I could I was burping solvent all night and much of the following morning. Spent hours with sensory memory yanking me back to the wood-stained sea-unworthy rowboat my brother, my dad and I took out on ill-advised Gulf Island fishing expeditions when we were kids. All we ever caught was kelp and, once, a dogfish, but we more than made up for it with Rip-L chip consumption.

I made a point of disclosing all death assays to my psychiatrist—because what's the point, really, of voluntary psychotherapy if you bullshit your way through it? He in turn was very tolerant of my continued efforts to undermine his Sisyphean work. He did ask, though, that out of courtesy I give him a head's up when I bought toxic substances at the hardware store, rather than after ingesting and regurgitating them. I'm not sure this was helpful, however:

"Do you still have that jug of antifreeze in your closet?"

"Yeah."

"After I told you to get rid of it?"

"Yeah."

"Why?"

"It makes me feel better to have it around. Like, in case I need it."

" . . ."

Technically, the paint-thinner incident resulted in my going to hospital but I tell myself it doesn't count because I went of my own accord, as an outpatient and a horrible liar, after e-mailing my psychiatrist who urged me to call poison control. Which I did, the following morning, traces of solvent lingering at the back of my throat. The voice on the other end freaked me out by demanding my name and contact info, which makes sense if you want poison control to save your life but is terrifying if you just tried to kill yourself and don't want anyone to find out and lock you up. The person urged me to get checked out in case the vomiting rerouted any solvent to my lungs where it would eat away at my alveoli, causing a fun kind of chemical pneumonia. I acquiesced, reluctantly. Partly because I was scared for my lungs but mostly because the poison control person now had my name and contact details and I was loath to get in trouble. I tried to appear nonchalant in hospital, which is hard to do when you're waiting in emerg with the non-emerg patients, driven hypochondriac by the sniffles of others.

The scan results were fine.

"You have scoliosis," the medical technician noted, eyeing the image.

"Yes, I'm aware. Thanks."

(Pro-tip: If you're going to say you "accidentally" swallowed a bunch of paint thinner—"'Ingested'? Do you mean you inhaled it?" "No, I mean ingested"—at least come up with a half-decent reason you had it around. And why it was in a glass or mug or thermos or some other container a reasonable person might accidentally drink out of. And remember that reason long enough to get out of the hospital.)

Things might have gotten weird if the solvent had done any measurable damage: questions would have been asked for which I had no truthful answers. But I was fine, my lungs looked fine. I went home and tried to reconcile myself with the prospect of remaining alive.

What do you do while waiting to die? Read, or try to. You want so badly for it to end this way—apartment clean, phone off, sitting on your bed, book in your lap, glancing out the window onto light and sun and life below. But you're impatient, easily bored: tough to lose yourself in fiction while anticipating a fatal hemorrhage. Less than an hour after ingesting fifty thousand milligrams of Aspirin, your first serious suicide attempt in years, you give up; your appetite for waiting wanes to a sliver, disappears. Self-discipline dissolved, you rise from bed, unlock your laptop, turn phone back on. Email your doctor, poor fucker, because you feel he should know and because in the vacuum of a botched attempt at death you crave even the rotest response. Call a friend, intrude on his workday, cause distress to someone you love because you need so badly to hear someone's voice, hear someone say, "I'm glad you're alive." Compound that distress by refusing to go to hospital to get your blood checked or stomach pumped.

"I'm fine."

"But what if you're not?"

"But I am."

"What if you pass out and don't wake up?"

So be it, you don't say. So much the better. You don't pass out. The acid roils your bloodstream, rings in your ears, distorts your aural world so for the next twenty-four hours everything sounds underwater. You hold your nose and blow as though your blocked-cochlea feeling is an altitudinal problem and not a drug-induced hearing loss. You lie on your side in a chill sweat, swept with nausea, a thrumming ache behind your eyes that finally abates and leaves you drained. The ringing persists. But you don't pass out. You still don't die.

I was abashed at how stereotypically girly all my attempts were: Women tend to go for poisoning, as noted; sometimes suffocation; men shoot themselves or hang themselves or jump from high places. Twice a day, on my bike ride to and from Global News, where I was now working, I traversed a pair of bridges. Each time I eyed their edges, trying to calculate whether they were high enough for a jump to guarantee death. I expended brainpower wondering how to ensure I'd hit the ground headfirst; it'd be just like me to klutzily fall wrong and survive, badly injured. My depth perception and distance estimation is awful. And I am paralytically afraid of jumping from heights—cliff-jumping with cousins from a handful of metres above water was enough to freak me out.

In the seven years following my first suicide attempt I moved apartments once, changed jobs twice and tried to end my life at least half a dozen times, depending what you count as a discrete attempt. Each suicide attempt made me more reluctant to try again not because I didn't want to die but because I couldn't stand the emotional letdown of thinking it was all finally over only to realize it wasn't.

I started wondering whether I really wanted to die badly enough, or whether I just kept punking myself. But the desire didn't dissipate.

7

Know Thine Enemy

I procrastinate the hell out of everything imaginable. So maybe it's no surprise I let my grandmother's exhortations to write a book percolate for years without doing much about it. But I found myself continually, repeatedly, compulsively pulling out a notebook or opening a Word document and scrawling misery a few words and snatches at a time, often from bed when I was unable to sleep or unable to emerge. I began to read everything about depression and suicide that I could lay my hands on and it wasn't enough: there was a gap in the discourse between redemptive narratives and anti-psychiatry polemics and academic screeds. And found that my experience, and that of many others, falls into that wide gap.

So I started making calls—just tentatively, because I had no idea what I was doing, and because I had (and was desperately clinging to) a day job. But I couldn't not: surely someone could shed light on this despair that buried me.

I reached out to Madhukar Trivedi, the founding Director of the Center for Depression Research and Clinical Care at the University of Texas Southwestern. He's in the midst of a decade-long study of two thousand depressed people, tracking numerous clinical, biological, sociodemographic variables and outcomes, and he helped walk me through how the disease first hits you. "Half the people who get depressed will get their first episode before the age of thirty," he tells me on the phone.[1] "They have a whole lifetime of suffering." He'd be the first to also tell you there is treatment out there now, and hope for better treatment soon—misery isn't a given. But that's a chilling thing to hear.

There is something perniciously unfair about a disease that strikes, as this one tends to, in early adulthood, just when you're supposed to be coming into yourself as a human being. You're poised within a world of opportunity—charging forward, flooded with plans and ideas and ambition—only to be trapped without warning in endless dark. That sense of purpose flickers back every now and then, only to be drowned out. *I can't. I can't.* It shafts your budding life partnerships, your education, your career.

Major depressive disorder starts, ostensibly, when clusters of symptoms cause serious, protracted impairment. How serious, how protracted does that impairment have to be for you to qualify as depressed? There's no surefire way to tell. It's easier to spot depression in its most awful extreme; far trickier to diagnose a much milder case.

"We dichotomize gradients."[2] Back in Toronto, where I live, Paul Kurdyak, a psychiatrist and the Medical Director of Performance Improvement at the Centre for Addiction and Mental Health (CAMH, familiarly known to locals as cam-aitch) has invited me to his office in an old brown-brick building close to the bustling streets of College and Spadina. The noise of the traffic and the late afternoon sunlight filters in through a west-facing window. A friendly man with dark brown hair who readily warms to his topic—I kept him talking in his office for hours and made him late, slightly, for a dinner—he balances clinical and research work and somehow manages to be insanely prolific and still piss off his own colleagues, as he did when he suggested there was little need for more psychiatrists—but a huge need for better care. I was drawn to his work on the burden of mental illness and showing the ways our system falls down on itself and fails its users, who if they're lucky wind up right back where they started.

"We have to draw a line somewhere," he says, "'cause that's just how clinical stuff works. We want to know if someone's depressed or not depressed, so we create this threshold." The worse your depression is, the more obvious it is you have it and the more effective the treatments tend to be. "There's a point at which antidepressants seem to have the biggest bang for their buck, relative to placebo, and it happens to be at the more severe end."

People in the fuzzy twilight between a mood disorder and a crappy mood state could be forgiven for thinking the whole thing's a sham. They may not have an illness and if they do, available treatments are unlikely to help as much as they might were their illness more severe. When detractors decry antidepressants as little better than placebo, this is the patient population they're talking about.

Who makes that call, dichotomizes that gradient? Usually the gatekeeper to care is your GP. I went to talk to Javed Alloo, a family doctor I reached through CAMH in my attempts to get a sense of what it's like dealing daily with mental illness and mentally ill patients as a non-specialist, a general practitioner. He is one of the few GPs who seeks out patients with often complex mental illness, rather than the reverse. Speaking in a North Toronto food court over the din of lunch-hour rush, and the melting gelato my questions prevented him from finishing, he explains how he deals with mental illness and how he demarcates between serious psychopathology and mild mental angst. The key is function and duration, he says: How long does the shittiness last, and to what degree does it stop you from doing the things you have to do to live and to make life worth living?

"If they're coming in to see me once every two weeks for fifteen minutes, and this is the worst expression of the anxiety in their life, their family's not complaining to them, it isn't stopping them from going out and doing stuff... then they don't need treatment. Obviously, it's not black and white. It's a spectrum. But the question is, at what point does it become dysfunctional?"[3]

. . .

IS DEPRESSION A NEW thing? An old thing? Is it becoming more prevalent, or are we just diagnosing it more readily? I discovered that while the more colourful and memorable depictions of mental illness tend to involve mania and psychosis, the Bible, Arab medicine, Greek mythology and centuries of European spiritual and pseudo-scientific record-keeping all make reference to enduring despair beyond any external trigger. First-century physician Ishaq ibn Imran called melancholy "that feeling of dejection and isolation which forms in the soul because of something which the patients think is real but which is in fact unreal."[4]

There's a real and widespread and understandable impression that depression is everywhere and increasing. In *The Noonday Demon*, the early twenty-first-century's seminal, masterfully written book on depression, Andrew Solomon describes the disorder as a malady profoundly exacerbated by modernity. Like skin cancer, he writes, "depression is a bodily affliction that has escalated in recent times for fairly specific reasons." Where a depleted ozone layer and carcinogenic soup have made skin cancer a much more common scourge, the strain of modernity—"the pace of life, the technological chaos of it, the alienation of people from one another, the breakdown of traditional family structures, the loneliness that is endemic, the failure of systems of belief"—has driven a growing number of people to depression.[5]

All these things affect us in as yet unknown ways, some of them bewilderingly new. But crippling despair divorced from reality, by whichever nomer you choose, has been associated with the stress of modernity for millennia. As far back as Aristotle, sociologist Andrew Scull writes, melancholia was associated with "outstanding accomplishment"; in the sixteenth and seventeenth centuries, "melancholia became something of a fashionable disorder among the cultivated classes, an affliction to which it appeared that the scholar and the man of genius were particularly prone." A century later, "nervous illness" became a marker of a civilized, refined individual or society, to which more supposedly primitive populations, busy with hunting and labouring and free of artifice and stress and the pursuit of excellence, were thought to be immune.[6] All of these are relatives of modern-day mood disorders. All have existed for millennia. All have been associated with modernity, to various degrees, since the concept of modernity existed. So that's not new.

There's no shortage of literature decrying a ballooning epidemic of mental illness and depression. But population studies indicate depression's prevalence is pretty steady, although its level varies. According to America's pre-eminent institution for mental health research, the National Institute of Mental Health (NIMH), at any given moment about 7 percent of the American population has depression,[7] which is about what depression's prevalence was when the National Comorbidity Survey was conducted in the early 1990s;[8] increasing use of antidepressants doesn't necessarily indicate an increase in the prevalence of depression or even its diagnosis.[9] World Health Organization statistics estimate prevalence at just under 5 percent globally—a number whose increase over time is in keeping with population growth and the growth in the number of older adults who are more likely to report prevalence.[10] Lifetime prevalence is closer to 17 percent, which means that almost one in five people will be plunged into despondent despair at some point in their lives.

The toll is high. The World Health Organization multiplied diseases' prevalence by the degree to which they wreck you and found depression to be the single largest contributor to disability in the world, swallowing up fifty million years lived with disability in 2015 alone.[11]

Suicide kills about 800,000 people a year globally but if you're being brutalized by depression, suicide isn't the only thing you're at higher risk of dying from. "Let's talk about heart disease. Let's talk about diabetes. Depression increases your risk of dying after you've survived a heart attack," Sarah Lisanby, head of translational research at NIMH in Maryland, says to me in one of multiple conversations we had as I fumbled my way through the field, and she was very understanding of my ignorance. Her job, largely, is to help translate esoteric, pie-in-the-sky cutting-edge research into new tools or insights that can be used in a doctor's, counsellor's or nurse's office. Depression, she says, "worsens not only your mental health, but also your physical health. And so even though neuropsychiatric disorders are the leading cause of disability, and this has been recognized, they're also the leading drivers of other causes of disability. . . . The impact of depression on your health goes beyond your brain."[12]

So why don't we take this illness more seriously? In part, perhaps, because depression, as a concept, has become a victim of its own success.

While pathological despair is hardly new, "depression" as a mood disorder really emerged in the middle decades of the twentieth century, as psychiatry sought to cast off both its asylum baggage and its pseudoscientific reputation: psychiatrists were to be considered "real" doctors, treating relatively "normal" people— not confined inside mental hospitals but walking around in the world. By 1980 "depression" went from being a word primarily associated with economic downturn to a disorder warranting an entry in that doorstopper of a mental illness dictionary, the *Diagnostic and Statistical Manual of Mental Disorders*, and became one of the most prevalent mental illnesses in the public discourse. Throughout the '70s and '80s, "popular magazine readers were increasingly told that depression was something that could affect them—and that rising rates of depression were a serious national problem," writes the psychiatrist and historian Laura Hirshbein (full disclosure: she's my cousin). Major depressive disorder was on the vanguard of illness as "consumer product"—something you could shop and self-improve your way out of. This persistent repetition in mainstream media made depression seem a common treatable condition but also made "depression" a word used colloquially to describe a general feeling of malaise.[13] This meant that having depression, the diagnosed illness, became easy to discount and easy to conflate with a ubiquitous human emotion that's unpleasant but hardly pathological.

That's one reason so many people fail to see depression for a real, diagnosed illness and instead see it as part of the normal spectrum of human emotion, creating a disorder where there is none, turning sick people into needy malingerers and those purporting to treat them into conniving charlatans. You can't do a lab test for depression—at least not yet—you just sniff out its presence based on squishily subjective variables. That makes it easier to discount but no less real or debilitating.

8
Checking Boxes

For millennia, we've recognized the difference between "normal" sadness and crippling despair. But we've never been good at delineating between the two. So the American Psychiatric Association's *Diagnostic and Statistical Manual* (*DSM*) defines depression by a list of symptoms rather than how it's caused. Zeroing in on the causes could have revolutionized our understanding and approach to depression, but we didn't because we've never known them. So you wind up with a morbid menu.[1] Do you feel "depressed" or irritable almost all the time, almost every day? Are you less interested in stuff you used to like? Have you gained or lost at least 5 percent of your body mass? Are you sleeping way less or way more? Are you way more active than usual or not active at all? Do you have no energy? Do you feel guilty or worthless? Are you having trouble concentrating? Do you want to kill yourself?

Officially, medically, if any insurer is going to pay for your drugs and your psychotherapy, you need to check off at least five of those nine boxes—and confirm that the symptoms in those boxes cause you "clinically significant distress or impairment in social, occupational, or other important areas of functioning."

First of all, the above violates what I would consider Nosology Rule Number One: Don't define something using the term you're defining. I have depression if I've been feeling "depressed" every day? Rookie tautological mistake, American Psychiatric Association.

Reading these criteria after my own diagnosis made me feel like a flounder—flattened, two-dimensional, bottom-feeding. They could apply to anyone and no one, I thought. You could have two people presenting almost entirely divergent symptoms and diagnose them with the same illness. Sometimes you successfully treat depression only to discover the things you considered symptoms are actually separate illnesses that persist on their own.

Anxiety, for example, can be either a symptom of depression or another illness altogether. The two frequently coexist. One distinguishing factor I learned while navigating my own neuroses is the nature of the worry: people with anxiety disorder tend to freak out about the future—what they want to do, what they're going to do, the infinite ways they could conceivably screw it up. If you're depressed, there isn't much of a future to worry about. People with depression-flavoured anxiety suffer crippling worry about the past, not despite our inability to change it but because of that. We ruminate endlessly about shit we did this morning or yesterday or last week or last year and how unforgivable it was and how everyone judged and continues to judge us and maybe we should ask them about it or no that would make it worse and what are all the possible ways they could have been upset about it and who are all the people they probably told? Angsty, ruminating moose.

The checklist is also incredibly reductive. The *DSM*'s authors boil down diagnosis of mental illness to something resembling an online quiz: Which Disney Princess Mental Disorder Are You? Online questionnaires like these do exist, with varying imprimaturs of medical legitimacy. You click through, answering questions about your levels of stress, anxiety, enervation, restlessness, appetite, mood. You're asked about your desire to die and when you click "hells, yes," a dialogue box pops up with a crisis line to call. I've clicked through a couple of those quizzes, both largely based on the kinds of questionnaires used to diagnose people in a clinical setting, both giving me that two-dimensional flounder feeling as I wondered what small changes to my answers I could make to get a different verdict.

Benoit Mulsant wants to see more of those quizzes. I'd sought him out at CAMH where he's Clinician Scientist, and among other things he's working on a way to diagnose and, hopefully, treat people in remote areas without access to psychiatric care. This matters: so much of mental health care is concentrated in big cities that it can be impossible for many people to access even a basic assessment that would allow you to figure out what care you need and whom you need it from. Crisis becomes the default. He likens his initiative to a "concierge" for mental health care: train someone to put patients through a standardized, symptom-based screening protocol designed to determine the severity of their illness, the kind of care they need, and then refer them to whomever's best and most accessibly positioned to provide that care. You don't actually diagnose and you don't need to be a physician or a nurse. You can administer the screening over the phone or online, so lack of physical access to a specialist doesn't preclude you from at least figuring out whoever's most likely to be able to help you, and then contacting that person directly to set something up.[2]

This "concierge" isn't widely available yet. For now, most formal diagnoses are still based on in-person interviews criticized by turns as too formulaic or too subjective. In his (fascinating) 2015 tome dedicated to a history of our conceptualization of mental illness, *Madness in Civilization,* Andrew Scull dismisses modern psychiatry's diagnostic methodology as "a 'tick the boxes' approach to diagnosis" that "eliminate[s] so far as is possible individual clinical judgment" and promotes "rapid, routine and replicable labelling."[3] But at the same time, I find, the *DSM* diagnoses rely overwhelmingly on a patient's ability to self-report and a physician's ability to recognize and identify nebulous characteristics that aren't nearly as easily categorized as the *DSM* would suggest. It doesn't help that people suffering from psychiatric illnesses often lack insight into their diseases as a result of the disease itself. As a doctor you need to assess a patient's mental state and read the bullshit between the lines. I don't doubt most clinicians have become adept at ferreting out the sick from the sad, malingerers from those trying to hide a more serious malaise. But a measure so subject to interpretation leaves a lotta room for error: When a doctor asks you if you've been feeling down, if you've lost interest in your daily activities, your definition of feeling down might differ from theirs. When a doctor asks if you've thought about killing yourself at all in the past two weeks, and you hesitate before saying no, how the doctor deals with that can change your diagnosis and course of treatment or lack thereof.

Given that this checklist definition was designed explicitly to avoid that awkward moment when two clinicians, ostensible experts in the same medical field, come to two different conclusions, it's ironic that it continues to happen.

I learned this firsthand when I found out after the fact that I'd been diagnosed with two different illnesses by two psychiatrists at the same institution within days of each other, and came close to being discharged immediately without any plan of care and without even being told what my diagnosis was.

The first psychiatrist who evaluated me—the one who earned my family's eternal dislike when she suggested we were all alcoholics— diagnosed me with borderline personality disorder. It's a diagnosis associated with impulsivity, emotional instability and interpersonal problems that include anything from a lack of empathy to emotional manipulation or separation anxiety. It's also characterized by almost dissociative self-harm, where you might surface afterward to wonder, "What just happened?" It's the kind of diagnosis that's easy enough to make, but has a much tougher time holding up to rigorous scrutiny. Knowing what I know now, I can understand why she'd slot someone who makes a serious suicide attempt and then insists everything's totally okay into that category.

And I get why that diagnosis was wrong. Problems I developed in relating to people, I learned all too well, came from the social withdrawal that's a common symptom of depression and turned me into an ornery unwilling hermit. My mercurial, erratic-seeming disposition came from the dizzying swing whenever my Super-Functional-Happy-Not-Depressed! coping-mechanism facade short-circuited to let my genuine unpalatable misery show through.

I didn't have a personality disorder; I was just desperately trying to swallow a disease that kept clawing its way to the surface.

I'm exceptionally lucky I got that second opinion, even though it meant those awful extra two weeks locked up, and lucky that the second opinion, the diagnosis of major depressive disorder, prevailed. Other people I've spoken with have been handed a multitude of divergent diagnoses and endured years or months of ineffectual treatment with unpleasant side effects before they and their doctors hit on something that worked. One acquaintance was told she had depression, then post-traumatic stress disorder plus anxiety. Decades later, after she'd constructed an identity for herself and spoke regularly on public forums about what it's like to battle mental illness, she was diagnosed with a personality disorder and the new, scary-sounding label sent her spiralling. The two of us pored over a binder of symptoms in an otherwise empty Japanese restaurant, by turns rationalizing, dismissing, making light of the label.

Chronic illness changes the way you see yourself—it outlasts jobs, homes, relationships. Even the flimsiest reification has power.

ELLIOT GOLDNER, FORMER director of Simon Fraser University's Centre for Applied Research in Mental Health & Addiction, started his career helping individuals struggling with mental illnesses and addiction in Vancouver's notorious Downtown Eastside. I was lucky enough to speak with him before his death in 2016. He told me over the phone that depression is perhaps better characterized as a bunch of different illnesses with sometimes similar symptoms: some people do get sick as a result of trauma—such external shocks as abuse, war, loss and sundered relationships, financial or professional disaster. Others don't have that tangible experiential trigger.[4]

That kind, my kind, the depression without an experiential trigger, is the kind we understand the least and that tends to be most resistant to treatment. It could be immunological; it could be parasitic; it could be genetic or epigenetic, or some weird combination of all or none of the above. Some prominent physicians have suggested depression results from unbalanced gastrointestinal microflora or a severe allergic reaction, or the common parasite *Toxoplasma gondii*—better known as the crazy cat lady parasite. (Sadly there's no evidence so far in favour of mood-stabilizing fecal transplants or antidepressant parasite exorcisms.)

Such subjectivity around diagnoses offers little comfort to anyone skeptical of the field's medical pedigree. And the critiques don't come from antipsychiatry activists alone: each update to the *DSM* unfolds like a backstabbing melodrama for geeky doctors, as titans of psychiatry denounce each other's approach to the foundation of diagnoses for the brainsick. Allen Frances, who co-authored the third edition back in the '80s, slammed the later versions as sloppy, secretive and potentially pathologizing normal behaviour such as grief.[5] Even the most prominent members of the psychiatric establishment have expressed skepticism bordering on blasphemy. "There's no reality" in the *DSM*'s diagnoses, then NIMH director Thomas Insel said shortly before the *DSM-5* came out in 2013. "These are just constructs. . . . We might have to stop using terms like depression or schizophrenia, because they are getting in our way, confusing things."[6]

The *DSM* has loomed large in the public and medical imagination, as a kind of bible and infallible conferrer of identity. But it's more useful, Thomas Insel advised me, to treat it as a dictionary rather than an encyclopedia.[7] This makes sense, but perhaps it's best to treat it as no more authoritative than its name suggests—a manual of diagnoses, a role it often plays now. It's possible, as much as psychiatry's categorizing authorities might hate to admit it, that our diagnostic designations are arbitrary enough to be unnecessary. Does it really matter if our best definitions of depression and other mood disorders are so nebulous as to lack meaning, as long as we can identify the people who need treatment and get them treatment that will alleviate suffering, make life worth living, without causing harm?

Maybe not. But, as I found out, we're pretty bad at treatment, too. Especially when it comes to the most fatal psychiatric phenomenon we're up against.

9

Suicide Blues

I never know what to say when people ask whether I've been thinking of killing myself "lately." Have you blinked lately? Longings for death are fleeting mosquitos that swarm—"Why am I alive?" "I want to die." "I should be dead"—dozens of times a day. They're compulsive obsessions, methods brainstormed at least once or twice daily, detailed plans hatched at least once a week. They're grisly nightly visions of accidents or homicides.

Suicidal ideations materialize like sexual fantasies: vivid, unbidden, distracting. Like a desiccating thirst pulling thoughts away from all else. The same anticipated relief. The same agony when that release proves out of reach. Blue balls, but for death.

I pictured in detail my bodily decomposition. What would go first? Would I stay fresh longer if I left the air conditioning on high? How long before the smell seeped into the apartment hallway, or through ventilation shafts into other apartments? My poor neighbours. I should send them flowers. I had an overwhelming desire to turn in my body and donate it wholesale. "I have *so many organs!*" I'd declare to anyone who'd listen, mutter to myself several times a day. This is just weird enough to sound like a sick joke to another human being but for me it never was: I was gobsmacked by my own wasteful monopoly on body parts. Dozens of people die every day awaiting organs, and here I was hogging so many of them—perfectly good pancreas, lungs, liver, kidneys that could save the lives of people who could then go on to win Nobel Prizes or solve refugee crises. That aspiration ran so deep, I felt cheated to discover you can only donate organs if you die while stabilized, on a ventilator—not if you're dead on arrival at a hospital. (If that fact doesn't sound devastating to you, you clearly don't dream up suicides designed so that no one will find you for at least thirty hours.)

Everything presents a path to death. I was disappointed to find nothing weight-bearing in my apartment to which I could fasten a ligature, but that didn't stop me from looping a stiffly knotted noose lengthwise around my door and trying to strangle myself with it. I peered over every ledge I got near and feverishly researched the toxicity and overdose potential of every drug I was prescribed.

When surgeons prescribed me Percocet in the wake of successive knee surgeries in 2017—meniscal arthroscopy followed four months later by a full-on ACL repair—all I could think of was the possibility of overdose. I said nothing when my first surgeon inadvertently wrote the same prescription twice: once before the procedure, and once afterward. The sixty 325-milligram pills I got each time felt like a precious gift, a personal hand grenade. I cursed my own weakness when I caved and took them one by one for actual post-surgery pain—wasting this precious resource on myself for no good reason.

But being swallowed by suicidality doesn't make all my actions actively self-destructive. I'm a hyper-defensive cyclist and do everything I can not to become roadkill, notwithstanding fantasies of being hit, dragged, pulled beneath a truck's undercarriage and crushed. I can't think of subways and streetcars without imagining throwing myself in front of one but my metro horror has me flattened against the wall in subway stations, as far from the tracks as I can get.

Every time I told my psychiatrist I'd come close to self-obliteration he'd ask, "What stopped you?" At first this sounded like a taunt: Why don't you kill yourself, already? If this were such a compelling obsession, why did I keep pussy-footing around it? His intent was not to goad me to suicide but to make me verbalize reasons for not dying.

Even once I'd recognized this, I still felt again and again like I was coming up short: I didn't feel I had a good enough reason for not having killed myself. I chickened out; I was tired; I didn't want to die in a messy apartment and didn't have the energy to clean it; I was scared of fucking up; I was scared of being found too soon. Other times, this line of questioning proved more illuminating: there were still questions I wanted to ask, things I wanted to do. Even half-assed senses of obligation—to work, to family, to someone I'd made plans to see—sometimes tipped the balance in favour of stasis over suicide. It's something I still ask myself accusatorily—What is *wrong* with you? Why haven't you killed yourself already?—but trying to elucidate good reasons for not being dead, writing them down for future reference, can be lifesaving.

Suicidality and curiosity are anathema to each other: You can't want to know things if you want to die. As long as I had questions I had reason to live, and when I was overwhelmed by a desire for death I could not begin to do the curious work that made life worth living. Unable then to conceive of an existence without suicidality, death is the best imaginable outcome.

On good days I could convince myself that I was no less worthy of life than any other organism. But even if I can convince myself that, objectively speaking, I have about as much justification in being alive as a blackfly, my brain flits to a much less easily dismissible fixation: What if I just don't *want* to be alive? What if I just don't like it? What if I'm just tired? And no matter how much psychotherapy you practise, that's tough to logic your way out of.

Pre-suicide priorities are nonsensical. I was most inclined to kill myself at times when I was confident no one would notice I was gone for a few days at least. Perhaps it's a testament to my sense of urgent desperation that, paradoxically, my most serious attempts were at inopportune moments—when I was supposed to be at work or had upcoming appointments. Even then, I convinced myself I had to at least make an effort to clean the apartment. More than once, this weird standard helped me put off an attempt because I lacked the energy to empty the garbage or clean the bathroom. A couple of times I made a point of buying non-perishable snacks and hard liquor for whomever I thought would have the shitty task of cleaning out my apartment after my death.

What does one wear to one's self-orchestrated death? Jeans, probably. And a T-shirt, but a clean one with no holes. A bra? If weeks- or months-old nail polish is chipping, do you peel it off or repaint it or does it not matter? Does comfort outweigh presentability, or is that dumb given that you're going to be beyond caring soon and this is the last impression loved ones will have of you? Showering and toothbrushing is non-negotiable, obviously. Floss and deodorant, less so. But should you make sure your hair dries well before you plan to go horizontal, lest you die with flattened curls hugging your scalp? What about moisturizing lotion for soon-to-be-dead dry skin?

You'd think, amid all this obsession, all these fevered compulsive plans, I'd leave room for a little consideration for the people I love, the people I harm through my self-destructive actions. Families, familial obligations, can be protective factors: for weeks one spring the only thing stopping me from killing myself was the fear it would ruin my brother's pending wedding. So why isn't this a deterrent all of the time? The answer's unflattering. I do think of my family and of the friends who count as family. I wish them joy and know I bring them profound concern. I hate myself for causing pain to the people I care about most, people who have the shitty luck of being close to me. But the guilt that engenders isn't enough to dispel suicidal ideation.

Sometimes because, as hideous as this sounds to say, being loved is a necessary prerequisite for wanting to live but it is not sufficient on its own. And sometimes guilt at what I do to my family foments my desire to die: I feel like a septic limb that must be cut off lest it kill the whole organism. A painful excision, but a necessary one.

You won't believe me but procrastination's the best suicide-prevention measure out there. If all else fails, if drugs and psycho-therapy and thought-record deconstructions all fall short and hope remains unreachable, the knowledge that you can still kill yourself tomorrow or next week or next month remains, perversely, the surest way to ensure you don't kill yourself right this second. In that same vein, the notion you've squandered all your chances, reduced everything to shit and will never have another shot at fixing your fuckups or escaping the shame they elicit, makes suicide seem a much more immediate imperative.

"People, they go back and forth between 'I don't know if I'm going to do this today; maybe next week.' But sometimes they're reassured that they have a solution, even though most of us rationally would say that's not a good solution," Jane Pearson, head of Adult Preventive Intervention and chair of the Suicide Research Consortium at the National Institute of Mental Health (NIMH), says to me. She was kind and helpful and followed up our phone conversation with a long email full of resources to check out and additional people to bug. She focuses on the catching-you-before-you-fall field of medicine: she studies how to stop suicides before they happen, whether from the emergency department or the community. "If you're collaborating and really trying to help somebody, you have to acknowledge that this is a solution they've come up with. And you can always say, 'I don't agree with that, but you got it. . . . In the meantime, let's see if we can generate other ideas. And help you find a life worth living.'"[1]

For fuck's sake, put it off. Postpone till tomorrow the self-obliteration you long for today.

It's excruciating to have someone you adore, someone whose suffering you loathe yourself for increasing, ask you to promise never to do the thing you spend 80 percent of your waking life thinking about. You say, "Promise me you'll never try again," and I, no matter how much I love you and want you to be happy and fulfilled and pain-free, think, "But what if I have to?"

The impulse to live and keep on living is one of the most basic of any organism. Self-extermination requires a force of will strong enough to override everything your body has evolved to do: survive. Vomiting, gag reflexes, pain thresholds, the need to keep breathing, a fear of heights or a thundering oncoming train—these all kick in involuntarily, bits of your nervous system at war with each other. There are also cultural and legal taboos that keep people from killing themselves. Most religions aren't cool with doing yourself in and sometimes hell can be an effective—albeit crappy, if you're suffering from self-blame already—deterrent. Attempting suicide was a crime in the UK until 1961;[2] in Canada, until 1972.[3] As recently as 2014, trying to kill yourself in India could've put you behind bars for a year, although like most penal sentences that doesn't appear to have been much of a deterrent: India's suicide rate grew from 10.9 per 100,000 in 2009 to 11.4 in 2013—an additional seven thousand people a year.[4]

What drives a person to that point?

There are countless factors at play but few are as esoteric as Hamlet's existential "To be or not to be." (Hamlet didn't off himself: Ophelia did.) The vast majority of suicides have one common element, and it isn't a detached intellectual conclusion as to the nature of being. Mental illness features prominently in 90 percent of cases for which coroners, medical examiners or forensic psychologists can determine a motive.[5] Regardless who you are or how you do it, if you kill yourself—or make an earnest effort to that effect—chances are compassionate, evidence-based care would have alleviated the awfulness you're dying to escape.

DEPRESSION'S THE MOST common mental illness giving rise to suicidal ideation but it's hardly the only one. There is a compelling argument for classifying suicidality as a distinct pathology— a disorder in its own right, rather than a symptom of something else. Maria Oquendo, past president of the American Psychiatric Association and the chair of psychiatry at the University of Pennsylvania's Perelman School of Medicine, has been lobbying for suicidality to have a section of its own in the next iteration of that thornily authoritative conferrer of legitimacy, the *Diagnostic and Statistical Manual*.

"Not everybody who is suicidal is depressed. And not everybody who is depressed is suicidal. But they're frequently comorbid pathologies." They're illnesses that go hand in hand, she tells me over the phone.[6] (I certainly see both in my own predicament.) Separating suicidality into its own category would, ideally, encourage the use of suicide-specific interventions or at least make it harder to ignore in the hope that by treating the mood disorder the desire to die will evaporate.

So if someone talks about feeling persistently down, for example, but mentions as they're leaving the doctor's office that they're thinking of killing themselves, having a separate diagnostic code for such suicidal ideation can remind the doctor to tackle it on its own. That would also make suicidal ideation in a patient or in the population easier to track: it would show up in the emergency department, for example, or in the coroner's office; it would make it easier for researchers to study the desire to die, to get a sense of how prevalent it is, where and among what populations.

Physicians and epidemiologists have been trying to uncover suicide risk factors: characteristics outside existing disorders that make people more likely to try to kill themselves. Hopelessness; an "over-general" memory that skips over specific details; hyperperfectionism; trouble solving problems; and a tendency toward black-and-white or all-or-nothing thinking are among them. Hopelessness certainly resonates for me: beyond sadness, self-loathing or any other negative emotional state, an absence of hope can be the most decisive thing propelling me to seek death. The shittier things get, the more the claustrophobic horizons of your world close in. There's no room for hope because there's no room for anything. So I confess it was news to me that not everyone with depression feels hopeless.

"Depressed people who still have hope tend not to become suicidal," says Tom Ellis, who when I spoke with him was the senior staff psychologist at the Houston-based Menninger Clinic and has been researching the differences between suicidal and non-suicidal mentally disordered people. "They come in and say, 'I'm going through a terrible patch. I'm hopeful, if I get treatment, I'll get better.' ... I would say the mere act of getting treatment means you have some hope."[7] (I agree and I disagree here. It's possible for me to have enough hope to take my meds but not enough not to try to kill myself.) A degree of psychological flexibility—the ability to notice your thoughts and feelings with a degree of circumspection, so they're *of* you but they're not *you*—can also be a protective factor against suicide. "So if I have a thought like, 'I'm no good,' I'm able to step back and say, 'That was just a thought that came up. It's not necessarily a fact ... nor is it necessarily going to be helpful, nor should I base my decisions, such as life or death, on the basis of a thought that comes up.'"

If eight hundred thousand people around the world kill themselves every year,[8] that means about twenty-two hundred a day, or three every two minutes. Statistically, two dozen people killed themselves in the time it took you to get out of bed, showered and caffeinated. Maybe forty-five during your commute to work; another ninety in the time you spent making dinner. Unless you, like me, take an eternity to do any of those things, if they happen at all. In which case, think of it this way: every time you mull killing yourself and manage to talk yourself down because you have more to do and more to ask of life, a handful of people have lost that internal wrenching wrestling match and ended it.

In Canada, where eleven people kill themselves daily,[9] you're almost ten times more likely to kill yourself than you are to be killed by someone else.[10] About 120 Americans kill themselves every day. Victims of America's gun epidemic are overwhelmingly suicides: Americans are more than twice as likely to die by their own hands as someone else's and almost twice as likely to shoot themselves to death than be shot to death by someone else.[11] If you die young, suicide's much more likely to be the cause: in 2016 it was the second-leading cause of death for Americans between ten and thirty-four years old.[12]

The vast majority of people who kill themselves are men—not because they're more likely to be depressed or suicidal but because they're more likely to choose lethal methods like guns. (Studies have found women actually make up the majority of people seen in emerg following suicide attempts.) Many, many more people try to kill themselves than actually do it—about half a million Americans are brought to emergency rooms every year after having tried to end their lives.[13]

Epidemiologists are leery of putting too much weight on sharp changes over short periods but America's spike in suicide appears too big to be a blip. The rate of people killing themselves in one of the most prosperous countries in the world jumped 33 percent in eighteen years, from 10.5 to 14 per 100,000.[14] It rose more for women than for men, which narrows the gap between the two but still leaves men four times more likely to kill themselves. The suicide rate among adolescent girls jumped the most, tripling—*tripling*—during that time period. (But keep in mind, the huge rate of change is influenced by a small denominator: 1.5 per 100,000 up from 0.5.)[15]

"When [the Centers for Disease Control] released their statistics of this increase between 1999 and 2014, people went, 'What?'" NIMH's Jane Pearson recalls. She just wishes there were more of that, more of a sustained palpable jolt in the public consciousness. "There was some recognition that this is a problem. But compared to other health problems, we don't have a Susan Komen foundation [one of the best-funded breast cancer organizations in the US], a big organization advocating for this."[16]

Her colleague Sarah Lisanby at NIMH—the head of translational medicine, in charge of morphing research into health interventions—doesn't know what's driving America's spike in suicides but she hopes the sharp jump will be a call to arms for the research and clinical communities. "We're making progress in terms of our neuroscientific understanding. We can translate that into public health impacts," she tells me, pointing to research into biomarkers and neurocircuitry that can mean new or better-informed treatments. "And we need to accelerate that pace of translation because people are dying."[17]

EVEN AS RATES rise, reality is likely worse: evidence indicates we're undercounting suicides by a significant amount—by as much as two-thirds, depending how you guesstimate. For one thing, despite the supposed decrease in shame in having a family member kill themselves, our persistent societal freak-out regarding suicide can make both relatives and authorities hesitant to classify deaths as such. There's a very high burden of proof required for coroners (usually in Canada) and medical examiners (in the United States) to classify a death as a suicide. There's rarely incontrovertible evidence: most people don't leave suicide notes and not everyone talks about killing themselves before killing themselves. Even if they had at some point in the past, how do you know this specific incident was a suicide? If someone is depressed, even suicidal, but also misuses drugs, how do you know for sure whether an overdose is purposeful? How do you know for sure whether a single-vehicle crash was careless driving or driven by a need for death? How can you be certain whether someone slipped or jumped?

You're more likely to find suicides when you look for them. And, much of the time, we don't. "The under-reporting of suicide is a recognized concern in Canada and internationally," reads a 2016 study by the Public Health Agency of Canada.[18] Suicide deaths are also examined a lot less closely, on average: about 55 percent of US suicide deaths get autopsied, compared to 92 percent of homicides.[19]

The more autopsies a county does, the more suicides it identifies, West Virginia University researcher Ian Rockett has found: if you spend more time investigating a death you're more likely to deem it intentional on the part of the deceased. I reached him by phone after reading some of his papers: he and his colleagues studied the rate of suicide classifications by county and found that the more detailed death certificates are, the more time coroners or medical examiners spend on them, the better-resourced they are to be able to do so, the greater that county's rate of deaths classified as suicides.[20] Another study, this one in Austria, found that the higher the autopsy rate, the higher the suicide rate: the more deaths you examine closely, the more of them you'll find to have been the result of tragic intentional self-harm, not tragic accident.

But we're doing fewer autopsies in Canada and the States, not more: the percent of deaths subject to autopsy in Canada dropped almost in half between 2000 and 2011—from 9.9 percent to 4.8, "further subjecting suicides to misclassification,"[21] the Canadian public health paper reads. In the US, autopsies dropped by more than 50 percent between 1972 and 2007.[22]

This has been a known issue for a while. The consequences of under-reporting extend beyond public health nerds who get off on accuracy. It suggests something is less of a problem than it is and therefore less deserving of our attention and our dollars. Which is convenient, given how icky it makes us feel in the first place. Finding fewer suicides can make it seem like suicide is less of an issue.[23]

"If you think about it, society hasn't been that invested in suicide prevention," Rockett points out. "If you more accurately portray the self-injury deaths and say, 'This is mental health,' there's potential for rather more resources to be directed toward the problem."[24] Take poisoning, where intent can be particularly tricky to divine: poisoning deaths classified as suicides dropped even as poisoning deaths classified as "undetermined intent" rose. Studies in both Canada[25] and the US[26] have found evidence suggesting it isn't just that people are making more unintentionally reckless decisions regarding what they smoke, snort, swallow, inject—we're actually misclassifying suicides as accidents. We know substance use increases your risk of suicide. But if you die thanks to a lethal amount of the substance you're misusing, your death is less likely to be classified as a suicide.[27]

Canada's Public Health Agency came to similar conclusions: overall suicide rates dropped. Suicide poisoning rates dropped.

Accidental poisoning deaths rose. Poisoning deaths of undetermined intent jumped by even more—almost 42 percent. The study estimated as much as 60 percent of suicides in 2011 were mistakenly labelled deaths of undetermined intent by self-poisoning. (The low end of that estimate is 15 percent, so take it with a bunch of salt. But it's still a double-digit underestimation.)[28]

Botched suicide attempts also go under-reported: many people who try to kill themselves either don't seek medical help or lie about why they are seeking it. I've done both those things. I'd do them again. As I've said, telling anyone you've tried to kill yourself, let alone someone you don't know, let alone someone who could suspend your right to freedom of movement, gives one enormous pause. (Not that telling someone you love is any easier.)

But take time to talk to people in hospital for near-fatal poisonings and it can be telling.

Infuriatingly but perhaps unsurprisingly, undercounting suicides, and therefore minimizing the self-destructive death toll and its magnitude as a public-health issue, is worse for marginalized populations.

The suicide rate for white Americans in 2016 was almost three times that of Black Americans.[29] "It didn't make a lot of sense to me," Rockett says. "I couldn't think of any other major cause of death where Blacks would have had an advantage." Fact is that non-white North Americans are less likely than white people to get any kind of care for their depression, much less care that meets evidence-based standards. Far fewer Black people who've killed themselves or may have killed themselves took antidepressants in the year before their death than their white counterparts which, given what we know about the role mental illness plays in the vast majority of suicides, suggests Black people are less likely than white people to get the psych treatment they need.[30]

And then the same marginalization that makes you less likely to get treatment also makes it less likely your death will be classified accurately, because lack of documented depression treatment leading up to your death makes coroners more likely to classify your death as being due to an "injury of undetermined intent."[31] Which means we're underestimating the toll this public health crisis takes on your community—and, therefore, the degree of need for prevention and interventions that could be directed toward it. Cascades of compounded marginalization. We probably aren't underestimating Black suicides by a factor of three, but maybe enough to be significant.

So what do you do with that?

Resources would help. More thorough—or at least more frequent—autopsies would help. Talking to people in ICUs would help. Lessening the need for absolute certainty in determining intent might also make classification both easier and more inclusive, albeit with somewhat broader definitions.

Ian Rockett would like to see a tweak in classification: instead of probing the recesses of someone's psyche at the moment of their death for a very specific kind of purpose—Was this overdose accidental or purposely suicidal or a combination of suicidality, self-destructive fatalism and a substance disorder?—medical examiners and epidemiologists could instead focus on the fact that the individual in question died by their own hand.[32] He says his preferred term is "drug self-intoxication." It combines what's now disaggregated into either "accidents," or "suicides," or "undetermined," excises intent and focuses on the fact that the dead person did this. In his ideal world, medical examiners would differentiate between licit and illicit drugs, tap into prescription drug monitoring systems to get a better sense of how the individual obtained the drugs that killed them.

He isn't suggesting eliminating entirely the category of accidental deaths. But he'd like to reverse the starting hypothesis, so that in order to rule something an accident you have to find evidence indicating an accident, rather than simply a lack of evidence indicating specific intent. Of course "there are deaths that are unintentional: a three-year-old gets into a cabinet and finds a pesticide." But "from an epidemiological standpoint, we want to approach things differently."

• • •

ONE WAY TO get at someone's intent at the moment of death is the psychological autopsy—where you trace back in time to get a sense of what was going through someone's mind and whether they wanted to die. At Ian Rockett's suggestion I called up Los Angeles forensic psychologist Michael Peck, who compares his psychological autopsies to background checks: "You interview people who knew the deceased. You find out what their life was like, what their last two weeks were like, who they talked to, what they did, what they didn't do. And you examine the details of the death method."[33] Some methods of death make it easier to suss out intent than others: a gun to the head is obvious; a gun to the chest is a little more complicated—could have been a cleaning accident. An overdose can be even tougher to suss out, depending what the person took and how much of it and whether this was something they had been prescribed for a legitimate purpose. If a person swims too far out and drowns, determining intent could rest on their swimming abilities, their mood or emotions leading up to death. Peck classifies some things as "sub-intentional suicides"—a single-person car crash, for example. "Even hanging deaths have been equivocal," he says. It could have been autoerotic asphyxiation gone awry. "The main way to get the intent is to interview the survivors of the deceased. It could be schoolteachers, it could be family members, it could be workplace friends. And try to get a picture of the last week or two, what was going on with them."

Even an unclear picture, a lack of contact with other people in the days or weeks before death, can itself be telling. "Most people tend to be surprised by the suicide. But as they're talking to someone like myself about it later on, it turns out they had more information than they knew they had. They saw things but never put it together." I've heard these kinds of rear-view mirror insights from the loved ones of a suicide victim and they are heartbreaking.

Peck tells me he gets a fair bit of pushback from people, especially those closest to the deceased, who often refuse to believe their loved one ended their own life. And there's more pushback if the person's young. "They usually say, 'Oh no, it couldn't be suicide. It's impossible.' . . . Our job would not be to convince them. Our job would be to give them information."

Sometimes there are psychiatric diagnoses in a person's past. But he won't fill in the blanks if there aren't—he doesn't try to diagnose the person postmortem. But he's unwound enough suicides after the fact to get a good sense of the most common precursors: social withdrawal and increased substance consumption—usually alcohol.

Michael Peck harks back to the halcyon days, decades ago, when there was the will to put time and money into proper psychological autopsies by trained professionals. Since then, he's seen policymakers' interest in suicide and such labour-intensive postmortem investigations come and go like loud music and big hair. "It costs money. So there has to be somebody willing to pay for it."

In the meantime there's the pressing question: What do you do while the suicidal person is still alive?

10

Getting in Trouble

It took almost four years before I got myself in trouble again. Spring of 2015. I was twenty-eight.

This is how it begins: Can't wake up. Can't get out of bed. Can't escape my personal infinite void. Can't shake off the oppressive weight that beggars verbalizing. I spend most of the day (Thursday) in a semi-conscious haze and by the time I get vertical I am convinced: I have to die. I can't countenance the prospect of more days like this, lost to uselessness and sweaty bedsheets.

There were window cleaners on my side of the building that day, and their presence added abstractly to my shame at the unmade bed, the papers scattered everywhere, the dishes lurking in the sink: I never draw my blinds, figuring I'm too high up in a neighbourhood with too few tall buildings to bother. But now I did, and eavesdropped on the faceless male voices whose language (Portuguese?) I didn't understand on the other side of my window. After they moved on to the floor above mine the twisting rope securing their scaffold remained, grey snaked with threads of pink and yellow tautly bifurcating the skyline. And I was propelled, by imperative, to action.

I cleaned the apartment, took out the trash, recycling, compost. Paid outstanding bills. Cancelled via email a Friday morning doctor's appointment and plans to watch a documentary with a friend that evening. Then I swallowed all the Parnate, my antidepressant, that I could handle.

Hundreds of those lovely circular scarlet pills tipped into my palms and tossed to the back of my throat. I'd just refilled my prescription and had at least six weeks on hand—about 4.2 grams of active ingredient. My gag reflex rebelled before I'd emptied the last pill bottle but I took enough—at least 3 grams—to comprise what should have been a lethal dose. Or so the papers I'd found online suggested. By this point I was being prescribed such a high dose, I'd developed a freakish tolerance for the drug.

For a minute or two I felt great. Surprisingly great. Like all conventional antidepressants, Parnate doesn't have an immediate effect and isn't supposed to. But I'd taken a monster amount and got a momentary high out of it. That didn't last long. I felt very awful very quickly. Dizzy and nauseous and trembly, unable to focus on any of the fiction I'd assembled by my bed to kill time. I breathed through my nose and swallowed repeatedly to keep sloshing stomach contents from rising to greet my upper esophagus. I tried to focus my unravelling attention on the window-cleaners' rope outside my window; on the labels on the world map on the opposite wall.

It was the questions that did it. The dumbest questions popped into my flailing mind—about labour rights and protections for people working on high-rise scaffolding; the places I'd never visited; the narrative arc of the book I'd just started (*Dust*, by Yvonne Adhiambo Owuor. A great read, if tough to follow while drug-addled). These were questions I wanted to be alive to ask. It's a curious revelation—like getting a second wind when you're about to collapse, combined with the sense of almost locking yourself out of the house. I wasn't happy. I wasn't hopeful. But I wanted to know things I didn't yet know.

I rocketed to the bathroom, watery Parnate filling the toilet with vivid fuchsia. I had the sudden urge to take a photo, willed myself to grab my camera on the other side of the apartment. But I wasn't moving. It didn't feel like I was having trouble moving. I just wasn't moving. Noticed from a distance that, as I washed my hands and face and tried to brush my teeth, I couldn't stop shaking. I'd grown used to antidepressants giving me microtremors. But these were not micro. I gripped or leaned against the white buzzing counter, unworried and unthinking.

Time passed faster than it should have. I retrieved my phone and watched the minutes tick by and battery drop one percentage point at a time. Exchanged texts with the friend I was supposed to meet, who'd kept my ticket, who urged me to cab it to the movie theatre. I registered detachedly how slow I was to dredge up words, how uncoordinated my fingers. I switched to a more predictive text input method on my phone only to find myself transfixed for ten, fifteen, twenty minutes at a time by the options it suggested. What did I want to say? The conversation did not go far. I wrote "sorry" a lot. By now it was late. Or dark, anyway. I knew I should email my psychiatrist, whose appointment I'd cancelled, but couldn't unlock my laptop. Had my password changed? Had I forgotten it? Even then, it did not occur to me that I was just messily mashing the keyboard, fingers like hot dogs.

I was intermittently awake for much of the night. I couldn't figure out why the city lights outside had all turned deep red, then green hours later. My eyes ached. There was still a delirium-inducing amount of neurotransmitter bouncing around synaptic clefts in every part of my body, from brain to gastrointestinal tract.

The next fourteen hours are fuzzy. When I wasn't asleep I sleep-walked or went dazed through drunken motions. I only registered efforts to reach me enough to avoid them. During a moment of semi-consciousness I tried to respond to a text from my sister, who'd asked me to check out an apartment for her that weekend. Typed garbled nonsense. Much later I was shocked to find photos with that day's timestamp on my camera's memory card, which means at some point I must have gotten up to shoot the view from my bedroom window.

That evening: more knocking, which I ignored. But then I heard keys rattling in the door as it swung open.

I remember the desperate dismay I felt as I leapt out of bed, half-dressed, and registered the pair of paramedics and the superintendent who'd let them in. I tried to piece together who had sent them. I willed my facial muscles and vocal chords to form words that would somehow compel them to go away and leave me alone. But I couldn't.

There's a disorienting panic at the sudden inability to communicate, like stepping forward and finding only air where ground should be. Whatever I did or didn't say was enough to convince them I should be hospitalized. I can't remember what I grabbed as they ushered me out the door but I remember going to grab a book when they stopped me.

"You won't need a book."

Lie. Boldfaced lie. But I was in no position to argue and lacked the motor skills to smuggle out reading material.

I couldn't tell you how I teleported to the ambulance—I mean, I assume I stood in the elevator, walked across the lobby and out the door, but I may as well have choppered out of there for all I know.

And then there I was. Back in the psych emerg at St. Joe's—fluorescent beige assaulting my eyes, plasticky chairs stiff and sticky against my limbs, cloaked again in mortification, my poor cousin summoned by family bat signal to my side. Humiliating memories of being instructed to pee in a cup but being too drugged up to do so or to communicate my inability to do so; of getting my period in the crisis ward (do not, ever, get your period in the crisis ward) and forgetting the word for "tampon." Then, several erased hours later, the sinking déjà vu of awaking in an ICU bed, be-gowned and strapped to IVs. My family flown in, again, freaked and teary but stoic and so goddamn loving I could not deal.

Failed suicides are not fun for emergency health workers, but I was an especially weird case. I remember having to get my blood work done a second time because apparently my circulatory, respiratory, nervous systems were functioning better than they should have been for someone with that much tranylcypromine inside her. At some point a physician returned with a scan of my brain (don't ask me when in the previous fourteen hours that happened; I've no clue) asking if I'd had a stroke. It took a bit of back and forth for them to confirm that this scar tissue was, indeed, a relic of my first suicide attempt, my pal antifreeze.

The choking guilt of causing pain to those you love, of betraying the trust of health practitioners who let you remain an outpatient and fill a month-long prescription, is only compounded by repetition. Shuffling from the intensive care unit to the short-stay psych ward is worse the second time around. You know what you're facing and you know you should know better. I was greeted by rueful nurses who remembered me from forty-four months earlier; I pretended I wasn't such a space cadet as not to remember them.

No matter how nice you are and no matter whom you sweet-talk, if you've just tried to kill yourself you're certifiable.

You'd think I'd be used to this but to have my craziness once again negate my freedom of movement was tough to bear. In no small part because the rules had changed thanks to an uptick in elopees and a couple of high-profile, outcry-provoking suicides in the region by inpatients who'd supposedly been under intensive psychiatric observation. I couldn't wear grown-up-person clothes. I couldn't leave the small windowless ward, not even with a chaperone. Again, I understand the public health concerns at the prospect of people like me doing rash things while in care. But even inmates in solitary confinement are entitled to an hour of fresh air a day. (They rarely get it in any meaningful way, and that's unconscionable. But still.)

I somehow prevailed on the empathic staff psychiatrist on duty that weekend to allow me off the Form, to stay as a voluntary inpatient in the short-term psych ward. I cannot adequately express the degree to which this simple act ameliorated my life in the immediate term.

Back to the psych ward. You know the drill. Sleeplessness that defied the earplugs and meditation apps the nurses gave me. Three tasteless mushy meals a day that I pushed around my tray while engaging in reluctant fragmented conversation with my fellow inmates.

I was more honest with my kind health practitioner interrogators this time around: I knew myself better and wasn't as desperate to prove my sanity. My expectations were low—I knew better than to expect any quick fixes—and I genuinely tried to engage in whatever treatment was put before me. I also got to know these nurses and social workers better. Talked with them about their lives, their hobbies, their teens' growing pains, adopted children, mixed-race families, workplace politics. Most had been propelled into the field by personal confrontations with mental illness, but their career choice still astonishes me. I implored trainee residents rotating through my ward to stick with this specialization. That weird plea from an oversolicitous mental patient could well have had the opposite effect.

My psych ward cohabitants were much more diverse this time around. A young Black woman who donned her hijab as soon as she graduated from hospital gown to real clothes—imagine being told you're too crazy for your articles of faith—asked which way was east so she could pray. It took a nurse and me a minute or two to figure it out; this would have been easier if we'd had *windows in the ward*, dammit. I was no longer the youngest one there. A lanky, sallow young man who worked airport security had checked himself in when his death obsession overpowered him. He was terrified he'd be fired for taking too many sick days. Another man, in his mid-twenties, had been arrested at the train tracks where he was prowling and preparing to throw himself in front of a locomotive. He was charged with trespassing (criminalizing suicidality seems like a great idea, right?) and had to call his parole officer from the patient landline on the counter. He read thick books on computer programming in between bouts of electroconvulsive therapy. They'd wheel him in afterward in a wheelchair and he'd be sleepy, slow, forgetful for a day or two. I don't know if the treatments did their job. I don't know what happened to the trespassing charge.

I felt I'd aged much more than the three-and-a-half years since my last inpatient stint. I felt decades older than the young girls in their early twenties brought sobbing into the ward by grimly desperate families, girls who snapped at the nurses and sequestered themselves in the dim behind bedside curtains. I was suddenly the most experienced person in the ward, the one who knew the rules for different forms, knew how often the psychiatrist would come and how much face time you could expect to get.

And my family was there. Again. I marinated in useless post-facto guilt. They brought me snacks and news from the outside world—there had been a major boxing match that week; apparently the domestic abuser won. We cackled too loudly, joked inappropriately, read aloud from newspapers and made each other guess which headlines were real and which we'd invented. Another lovely thing about not being formally committed (thanks to that kindly psychiatrist) was not needing them to chaperone me everywhere. I could leave the hospital for brief stints and meet them for dinner or whatever like a normal human being. I was irrationally worried that someone from work would see me and call me out for not really being sick. But it felt so great to locomote independently.

Let the record show I was a model patient. I changed my sheets daily from the linen stacked on shelves by the washroom. I made small talk and acted like a person who enjoys other people. I tried to explain ward protocol to the uninitiated. I loaned books destined never to be returned. I could have signed myself out but stayed for as long as the staff psychiatrist recommended, even when it meant sticking around an extra weekend so I could get a more complete assessment the following Monday. Before taking off I even did a weird mock assessment with a bunch of friendly, wide-eyed doctors in training, during which I told the truth to the best of my ability despite feeling I was either too crazy or not crazy enough to be a representative sample. I've no idea if I helped or hindered their training but I got a coffee shop gift card out of it, so I win.

. . .

TAKING DRUGS SUCKS but my god, withdrawing from them is worse.

My psychiatrist decided my Parnate overdose indicated it was time to wean me off Parnate. So he prescribed an antipsychotic olanzapine bridge during the weeks-long washout period before moving me to a new drug (you've gotta wait for the old one to clear out); and that wasn't enough to keep me from being an emotional train wreck after leaving hospital. And, as tends to be the case in downward spirals, my cognition was crap. It didn't even occur to me to attribute this total garbage feeling to antidepressant withdrawal until someone else pointed it out. I was on vacation spending a few days at my friend Omar's place in Portland, Oregon, so irrationally despondent that I convinced myself I needed to leave so as not to inflict my despair on him. He stopped me, and on an aimless impromptu sightseeing drive that would include visiting a Vietnam War memorial asked me what was up.

"I don't *know*."

"Are you still seeing your doctor guy?"

"Yeah. . . ."

"Have you switched up your meds at all?"

"Yeah, I'm off the stuff I was on before but I have this weird in-between period before I can start new stuff, because serotonin—"

"Okay yeah, I think we've figured out the problem here."

". . ."

So that was a fun time. I had a similar experience while chasing Hurricane (later downgraded to tropical depression) Florence in North Carolina for Reuters in 2018. When my editors asked me to extend my stay I of course acquiesced, even though it meant I would run out of meds—I'd brought just enough to get me through the week as planned. I tried getting my doctor to call a North Carolina pharmacy, I walked into an urgent care clinic, I got my sister to try to mail meds but still ended up sitting shaking in the Raleigh airport, three days into going unwillingly cold turkey. Thankfully getting back on the meds swiftly recalibrated my neurochemical equilib-rium. But fuck.

Seriously, no matter how useless your drugs are (or seem) I highly recommend talking to your doctor before you go rogue and stop taking them. Your synaptic clefts will thank me.

PART II

TREATMENT ATTEMPTS

11

A Pill-Popping Parade

Turns out I have a great metabolism for toxins. So says my psychiatrist—the second one I saw in hospital, the deep-voiced runner and motorcyclist who agreed to take me on as an outpatient and has seen me regularly, dealing with my freak-outs, meltdowns and cynicism, for the past seven years—when he ups the dosage of my latest drug for the umpteenth time. This freakish toxin tolerance does not apply to food or to booze, unfortunately. But fill me with neurotransmitter-altering substances notorious for wreaking havoc on gastrointestinal tracts and sundry endocrine mechanics, and they zip unnoticed through my bloodstream.

I am a reluctant pill-popper. I started out militantly opposed to pharmacologic treatment. I'd heard and believed all the horror stories: that these drugs wouldn't work but would have devastating side effects; that they'd turn me into a different person; that they'd leave me neither happy nor miserable but merely an unfeeling automaton lost in a neutralizing fog. That they'd backfire and just make me want to kill myself even more.

My psychiatrist had little sympathy for these fears. How could I claim to want to get better—as I had, vehemently, to get him and my parents and everyone else off my back and to get out of psych-ward custody and back to work—if I was unwilling to try even the most basic meds?

So, okay, fine, I swallowed my objections and a tiny daily pill in the hopes of being set free of the locked ward.

With the benefit of hindsight, I would like to note that my acquiescence was influenced by substantial pressure: I wanted to leave the hospital; leaving hospital required a doctor's approval. I wanted to go back to work; my workplace wanted a doctor's approval. My doctor wanted me on meds. Of course I went on meds. Years later I think this was the right move but I maybe made it for not the best reasons.

So I launched myself onto the psychopharmacological merry-go-round.

I started on a tiny dose of a little white pill called Cipralex (the brand name for escitalopram). It's one of the newer drugs in a group known as selective serotonin reuptake inhibitors (SSRIs—brace yourself for a whack of acronyms) and their great trick is supposed to be keeping more serotonin bouncing around your synaptic clefts. Like most of the drugs I took, Cipralex has been accused of being a "me-too" antidepressant,[1] where a tiny molecular alteration to an existing compound used for the same purpose does little to make it more efficacious but, once approved, allows drug companies to establish or preserve a lucrative patent while competing in the same therapeutic space.[2]

For a long time serotonin was believed to be The Answer—the key to depression, mood regulation and happiness. It's basically a chemical messenger your body produces that carries signals from one neuron to another, from your brain to your gut to your blood. Selective serotonin reuptake inhibitors are supposed to selectively keep the serotonin bouncing about in the gaps between neurons, the synaptic clefts, stopping it from being reabsorbed (that's the reuptake) back into the neuron. Instead, the serotonin just keeps making you happy as it bounces around for extended periods of time in those clefts. In theory, anyway.

Then it was thought The Answer was serotonin along with a couple of other neurotransmitters: dopamine and norepinephrine. They, too, are chemical messengers, bouncing around your synaptic clefts between neurons before being sucked in, reconstituted and shot back out again.

But the truth is, these popular explanations of antidepressant mechanisms are wrong. In theory, depression negates happiness; antidepressants alleviate depression symptoms; antidepressants increase concentration of serotonin, dopamine and their chemical cousins; ergo serotonin and dopamine create happiness. Wrong. I spent years picturing the synaptic cleft as pinball machine, reuptake inhibitors as "ball lock" mechanisms allowing a player with my cruddy emotional reflexes to keep more balls active, more happy lights flashing, more digital points accumulating.

Doesn't work that way. Neurotransmitters are not discrete silvery balls but molecular combinations of a series of smaller balls that keep getting broken down and put back together once they get yanked back into the neuron. And as I was to learn, increasing concentrations of one or all of those neurotransmitters does not guarantee happiness or even the alleviation of despair.

So our decades-old assumptions about, first, what those neurotransmitters do for us and, second, what drugs do to those neurotransmitters, are primitive at best. Large amounts of the bodily chemicals that psychiatric drugs target exist outside of the brain— they proliferate in your stomach, intestines, platelets. Turns out, we have only the vaguest idea how they work on a biochemical level, and no clue how that biochemical reaction changes your mood.

The depth of that uncertainty is destabilizing in the extreme when you're depending on those drugs to keep you going. So I can understand the allure of simple, wrong explanations. In the face of so much weird stuff going on in your brain, you fill in the gaps in comprehension however you can.

The first time I swallowed a single small elliptical white Cipralex pill, standing beside my curtained-off hospital bed, I was petrified, convinced it would brainwash me, rob me of personality. I sent a panicky idiotic text to a friend: "I'll love you even if this thing totally wrecks my brain forever, okay?"

I waited. It didn't. Apart from a little bit of jitters and a little bit of drowsiness, both of which soon dissipated, I experienced zero side effects from that first drug. This pattern repeated, more or less, with every drug I was prescribed: no seizures, no massive weight gain or loss, no loss of libido, no loss of self, no loss of emotional range, no worsening of suicidal thoughts, which I was learning to call by their more official-sounding name of suicidal ideation. Chronic lassitude and fatigue were, for me, more a familiar symptom of depression than a side effect of any new medication. Ditto sporadic insomnia, which for me seemed more a function of tightly wound anxiety than pharmacological intervention. Sure, there was wonkiness: some drugs made me trembly, some made me antsy, one made me sweaty; one made me dizzy if I rose from a chair too quickly right after increasing a dose; one blurred my vision (we rapidly decreased that dose); one made me sneeze endlessly; some made me nauseous, especially on an empty stomach, especially with espresso on an empty stomach, which makes for less than pleasant morning commutes. But that's par for the course when you bombard a GI tract with digestion-muscle-moving meds and nothing to digest.

Not all of those dodged bullets were as great as they sound: intensifying social withdrawal—a typical symptom of depression—meant I was going for weeks without interacting with anyone outside of work and psychiatric appointments and maybe family phone calls. I was certainly not banging anyone. Preserving one's sex drive is hardly a blessing when you're simultaneously suicidal and sexually frustrated.

And any advantage conferred by my lack of side effects was erased by my lack of any effects, period. I felt like I was popping sugar pills. My psychiatrist contended that the lack of improvement was at least partly in my head: that I'd have been far worse off—and may have killed myself for real—without that parade of meds. And he could be right. (His counterfactual's impossible to disprove, anyway.) There were certainly periods when things got better, or plateaued, and periods when they got worse, and it's possible my meds played a role in those shifts. It's also possible they didn't. But I wanted to feel *better*: not happiness or even an escape from despair but simply a consistent, propulsive sense of purpose. I need to keep getting up and out of bed and into the office in the morning.

Over the next seven years we experimented with fourteen different drugs in dozens of different combinations. As I write this we're considering others. We haven't yet found a combination that works.

We tried the circular lilac pills of bupropion, the generic version of Wellbutrin, which targets dopamine and norepinephrine. It was not until much later I learned Wellbutrin has become a common drug of misuse:[3] It produces a powerful high comparable to amphetamines and crack cocaine if you crush and then snort or inject it. Doing so can also produce gross, potentially fatal abscesses or blood clots or masses of dead tissue. Don't chance it. (That said, I have a couple dozen pills left lying around, if anyone wants to hit me up.)

We tried lithium, white and pale pink capsules. Popping lithium freaked me out at first—it's the one they give people with bipolar disorder, to balance the swing between manic highs and depressive lows, the one Claire Danes' bipolar character Carrie Mathison takes in *Homeland* to keep herself together. It's an effective mood stabilizer but long-term use can kick you in the kidneys if you aren't careful.[4] A friend in family medicine told me he had a patient whose bipolarity was so debilitating she'd been on high doses of lithium since early childhood. It regulated her mood but messed with her insides over time. The trade-off was worth it, my friend said, for the three decades of liveable existence. Suicidal ideation at least negates fear of terminal illness, which is a plus.

But more than kidney failure, what scared me was that being prescribed lithium proved I was even crazier than I thought.

"Are you sure I'm not bipolar?" I asked my psychiatrist for the zillionth time. "Are you *sure*?"

"You wish."

I just don't get the exuberant-invincible-impulsive-boundlessly energetic episodes characteristic of mania. That didn't stop me from periodically suspecting I'd experienced a manic or hypomanic episode. My psychiatrist raised his eyebrows at my descriptions of such brief, bizarre bouts of irrational motivation or well-being.

"Yeah, no, that's not mania. That's called feeling normal." The fleeting sense of being energized by, engaged in, hopeful about what I was doing felt so foreign I was sure it was symptomatic of another mental disorder.

Lithium's been used as a psychiatric medication for millennia. The mineral was isolated and defined in the mid-nineteenth century but its use goes as far back as the great Greek physician Galen, who got manic patients to bathe in and drink alkaline, likely lithium-containing, water.[5] But we don't really know what it does for people who aren't manic-depressive. We don't really know, on a molecular level, what lithium does, period.[6] But it is supposed to curb suicidal ideation, which in my case was a fairly urgent necessity.

We tried Cymbalta, olive green and navy blue, to inhibit my reuptake of serotonin and norepinephrine. By this time I'd become a reluctant expert at dry-swallowing handfuls of pills, throwing them to the back of my throat and swallow-shuddering, swinging my head side to side like a floppy-eared wet dog to encourage downward peristalsis.

We tried olanzapine, aka Zyprexa, an antipsychotic. It's a terrible thing to be told to take if you live in fear of losing your grip on reality. This fear dissipated with repetition, as I kept taking pills designed for different kinds of disorders than what I thought I was going through: studies have found various mood stabilizers, antipsychotics, anticonvulsants, anti-anxiety meds and other fun things can help alleviate treatment-resistant depression, especially when combined with a more conventional antidepressant.[7] And our ignorance of these drugs' biomechanisms is about equal, so why not?

That was when we tried Parnate, an old-school MAOI, a monoamine oxidase inhibitor, that seemed to be working until I tried to kill myself with it. Parnate, aka tranylcypromine, targets a different step in the same neurochemical pathway: it impedes the breakdown of all those neurotransmitters once they're sucked back into the neuron,[8] so instead of being taken apart and rebuilt in the neuron they just get shot back into the synapse to bounce around again like those happy-making pinballs.

I asked a med-school friend if he'd ever prescribed an MAOI.

"Of course not. I'm not a dinosaur."

MAOIs were popular in the 1950s and '60s. They worked well, by the flawed measures we have. But no one's prescribed them much since. There's so little demand for these drugs that the Quebec GlaxoSmithKline facility producing my Parnate put it on back order at one point, making it unobtainable for weeks and sending me into a minor panic, calling every pharmacist in the city seeking drugs. It led to surreal scenes that made filling a prescription resemble the world's most boring iteration of *The Wire*:

Man in white coat slides white bag across counter.

"Do you want to count that?"

Open the crinkling white paper, rip staple and reach inside to roll the cylindrical bottle of softly rattling pills out onto palm.

"Looks right. Thank you." Pause. "So . . . I can come back in three weeks for a refill?"

"Well, insurance usually prefers refilling at least two-thirds into dose, but that's four weeks' worth, so, yeah, I guess. . . ."

"I mean, will you have enough? Will you run out again?"

"Oh. Right. Yeah, should be fine. And . . ." —glances around—*"I know who'll have it. I'll hook you up."*

All this for a plastic container of crimson pills that'd be way easier to get if they had any street value whatsoever. The lack of demand isn't because MAOIs are less chemically efficacious than the various reuptake inhibitors that replaced them.[9] MAOIs are deemed too dangerous if you overdose, and possess so many unpleasant side effects, even if taken as directed, that patients just stop taking them. For me, this was the trembling- and vertigo-inducing drug. More troublesome were the nonsensical new dietary restrictions: MAOIs impede your body's ability to break down tyramine, found in a long list of foods from cheese to draught beer (but *not* bottled; don't ask me why) to miso and other fermented soy products to cured or smoked or pickled meats.

I cheated, of course. Usually because I forgot. And because cheese. And because on the rare occasion I'd meet friends at a pub, ordering bottled beer while everyone else sipped pints felt weird. Most of the time this illicit ingestion made no difference. But sporadically it gave me hours-long killer headaches, pain pulsating from somewhere beneath the front of my skull before eventually dissipating. Each time I vowed never again to eat whatever had so upset my wonky benighted internal chemistry—a pledge that lasted a day, maybe.

Doses went up when shit got rough or after I'd passed some invisible tolerance boundary and I took them as directed and prayed they worked with the same fervent hope you'd place in an amulet of dried goat testicles, if you could read peer-reviewed papers about the testicle-amulet's efficacy online and pose goat-testicle questions to the person who'd prescribed them to you.

But seriously: I believe in medicine and in scientific method; I gradually got better at sorting bullshit claims of causation from more believable ones; I got better at asking more informed nosy questions about effects and efficacy during my psychiatric appointments. But at the end of the day, health care relationships are predicated on trust—brain-health relationships overwhelmingly so. In part because all the things prescribed to me, all there was available to prescribe, did pretty much the same thing, on a biochemical level, as far as we know. And in part because the symptoms they were supposed to alleviate are so tough to measure, especially because depression's proclivity for seeing everything through shit-coloured glasses also applies to one's own prognosis. People with especially bad depression tend to be the last ones to realize they're getting better, but knowing that hardly helps. I had to believe each pharmacological adjustment would be the thing that tipped some imperceptible scale and took the draining effort out of the simplest tasks, leaving me energy left over for the projects meant to give life purpose.

My friend Omar called Parnate my hipster drug—"Really old-school; you've probably never heard of it." For a while my psychiatrist seemed to think it was working, till that aforementioned spectacular fuckup on my part eliminated it as an option.

We tried buspirone (Buspar), an anti-anxiety med.[10] And Zoloft, or sertraline, which targets serotonin (it was America's most-prescribed psychiatric drug in 2016).[11] We tried Lamictal (lamotrigine), an anticonvulsant with the delicious potential for eating flesh—a very rare, lurid, potentially lethal allergic reaction. Toxic epidermal necrolysis does pretty much exactly what its name suggests.[12] Watch out for painful red-purple rashes spreading from torso to face and limbs; for inflamed sores in your eyes, mouth, genitals. Skin and mucous membranes blister and peel away. If left untreated the disease can wreak deadly havoc on your internal organs. But to my dismay, no flesh-eating disease materialized; no skin sloughed off to reveal the oozing dermis I'd been promised. Perhaps not so coincidentally, I clawed lesions into my skin even more compulsively in the months following that disappointment, as though compensating for my lack of dermal necrosis.

My psychiatrist thought maybe trying a stimulant would ameliorate my paralytic enervation. So we tried the generic version of Adderall. Given Adderall's reputed popularity as a drug of misuse among overachieving students intent on pulling all-nighters, I assumed I'd pop a cerulean-blue, Dijon-yellow two-tone capsule and morph into a wicked-focused shark with a laser attached to my head. Not so much. I felt normal. Was able to work, which was great, but no better or more focused than before. No lasers. No searing propulsive purposeful energy. This was a letdown.

We tried Trintellix, one of the newest and not-yet-well-understood antidepressants out there,[13] but the pink egg-shaped pills did not seem to help any.

Then another new-ish drug, Pfizer's antipsychotic Zeldox (ziprasidone). Only the brand name was available. At this point I was uninsured and my drug bill topped $400 a month. I dipped into my savings and tried, with little success, to cut down my spending on necessities like food and books. For a while I was on an anti-psychotic (ziprasidone), an anticonvulsant (lamotrigine), an antidepressant (sertraline) and a mood stabilizer (lithium) all at once. I relied on my multicoloured, fourteen-compartment dosette to keep it all straight.

For all the potentially lethal things I put in my body on a daily basis, it's hilarious and not a little ironic that I remain alive. But it's grimly comforting to know my madcap psychopharmacological hopscotch is not outside the norm. There's been research support-ing the use of various drug combos as adjunctive treatments for depression that doesn't respond to conventional antidepressants right away, but it's a crapshoot determining which you should try and in what order.

This is true even for masters of the neuropharmacological craft.

Richard Friedman, the Director of Psychopharmacology at Weill Cornell Medical College in New York, does this for a living.[14] "Some [doctors] just clinically have a few they're used to using and they're comfortable with, and they try them, and you could say, 'Why are you using strategy A instead of B or C?' and the answer's not going to be 'Science.'" He's tasked with figuring out what alchemical medication cocktail to use on people who don't get better with the basic ones. (Andrew Solomon, the revered author of *The Noonday Demon*, told me he swears by Friedman's pharma-cological acumen.) Faced with a degree of treatment-resistant depression in a given patient, "I would give him something that, if they've had it in the past, worked if they've had prior episodes of depression. And, short of that, from a scientific point of view, you could take a coin out of your pocket and flip it."

Has he gotten better at this guessing game?

"I would like to say the answer to that is yes. If you asked me to prove it, I couldn't. So I'll say yes, but. I don't really know. Because this is not science. This is clinical gut feeling."

As few as one in four people start to feel better on the first antidepressant they try, if they take it as directed and stick with it for the six-plus weeks it'll take to kick in. That cumulative remission rate goes up to about 70 percent if you include people who go on to a second, third or fourth cocktail of drugs plus psychotherapy, with a smaller proportion of the remaining suckers getting better at each treatment step. The National Institute of Mental Health's Sequenced Treatment Alternatives to Relieve Depression Study (call it STAR*D if you wanna impress your psychiatrist friends) ran 3,671 depressed Americans through a flowchart of treatments. People who didn't respond to the first, second or third steps and continued on to Step 4 tended to be slightly poorer and older; they were more likely to be male, unemployed and uninsured. People whose depression had started before age eighteen and whose latest depressive episode has lasted for at least two years were also more likely to continue to Step 4.[15] Feels like I'm on Step 8,000.

So much for getting well. Staying well is another matter entirely.

Of all those people whose despair lifted on the first, second, third or fourth treatment combo they tried, almost half will be plunged back into despair, back to baseline within a year. "And then you're struggling to find out what is the next best treatment for them." The University of Texas Southwestern's Madhukar Trivedi is another master of his craft clearly distressed by the limitations of the field. "The more treatment steps you need to get better, the higher the relapse rate."[16]

In other words, the earlier your depression starts, the longer it lasts and the longer you wait to start treatment, the longer it will take for treatment to work and the more treatment combinations you'll need to try before something works. The longer your depression lasts and the more steps it takes for you to find something that works, the more likely it is you'll relapse in a year and end up right back where you started. The longer and deeper and more frequent your depressive episodes, the more likely they are to keep coming back as your habit-loving brain starts to think this is normal.

The need for swift, effective action on depression makes it all the more important to catch it early and makes our lack of effective, accessible treatment all the more inexcusable.

Even using the most optimistic efficacy estimate we're still left with about seven-million-odd North Americans enduring a chronic, debilitating illness and getting no lasting respite from any available treatment.

"There's still going to be a huge gap of unmet medical need that is just awful," says Steven Hyman, who heads the Harvard-MIT Broad Institute's Stanley Center for Psychiatric Research.[17] He's spent years wrestling with treatment options for mood disorders, or lack thereof. "Even those who don't kill themselves, their lives are very problematic. Because not only are they suffering but they are, I think we know by now, they're highly impaired."

(It's at this point in the interview I find myself at pains not to bellow, "I knowwwww, right?")

Given all that, is it any surprise that so few people suffering with depression take their drugs as directed? Even if they don't mess with your bodily functions, popping them daily for years on end with so little to show for it is really, really discouraging. Adherence rates in the medium term (three months from initial prescription) are about 40 percent, on average. By comparison, almost three-quarters of people with hypertension and two-thirds of people with type 2 diabetes take their meds as instructed at least 80 percent of the time.[18] This isn't because people with severe depression just aren't motivated enough to get better, although that's doubtless part of the issue: when severely depressed, it's impossible to get motivated enough to do much of anything. All too frequently, though, antidepressants' side effects are so intolerable they outweigh the drugs' (gradual, incremental) benefits. So people just stop taking them. The most common complaint is the havoc they wreak on your gastrointestinal tract, flooding it with neurotransmitters, increasing motility and making your gut all jumpy. That's why doctors recommend against ingesting these drugs on an empty stomach: a little substrate can give those muscles something to play with so they're not quite as cranky. Then you get anxiety, agitation, insomnia—also frequent antidepressant side effects, which is especially annoying because these tend to be either symptoms of depression or exacerbators of it.

But the one you'll hear about the most is sexual dysfunction. Because who wants that? What further proof do you need that psychiatry is an enemy of joy? These drugs can lower your libido, make penis-owners impotent, delay orgasm or make it unreachable altogether. We're not quite sure how this works; it may have something to do with receptors in your spinal cord.[19] Antidepressants' cockblock effect could be overblown, though: depression can do the same thing. (For this same reason, I'm personally skeptical of claims that antidepressants make you suicidal. It's akin to blaming chemotherapy for metastatic tumours, or lozenges for a sore throat. Just 'cause a treatment is inadequately efficacious doesn't mean it's responsible for symptoms of the illness it's supposed to treat. Antidepressants can, however, make you well enough to act on suicidal thoughts you lacked the energy and wherewithal to act on before, but which you were having anyway. Because life is a cruel trick.)

When every drug you take falls short of your desperate desire for remission, or when you simply get fed up with side-effect roulette, it's easy to think it doesn't matter whether you take the meds or not.

Wrong. Wrongety-wrong-wrong. I've had moments where I was convinced a drug was doing fuckall only for me to realize how much worse shit got when I was taken off it.

Just because something isn't nearly good enough doesn't make it entirely useless.

The ease with which antipsychiatry types use ignorance of how depression works and the limitations of existing treatments to bolster their arguments that the illness itself is a sham drives Madhukar Trivedi nuts. "I think that the efficacy challenges are real. We need to confess that. On the other hand, I can tell you that a lot of chronic medical diseases have the same efficacy challenges. We don't question the existence of those diseases. We become humbled by the outcomes. The jump in logic is remarkable—that because the efficacy is modest maybe it's not a real disease."

He sees two fundamental problems: A lack of information—people don't know what antidepressants can do, could do, probably won't do. And a lack of seriousness accorded to the condition they're supposed to ameliorate. "I still get asked questions about whether this is some kind of brain disorder." (For the record and the umpteenth time, he says, it is.)

There's evidence different kinds of treatment tend to work better when combined—drug plus psychotherapy is probably better than either in isolation; certain combinations of drugs may work differently on your brain; exercise can be a helpful adjunct to whatever else you've got going on (maybe something to do with those endorphins, or some other chemical reaction). But clinicians rarely coordinate them. "We should not rest on our laurels as soon as someone gets into remission. We need to think about what else needs to be done. . . . When you add those treatments that work potentially through a different brain mechanism, you get higher rates of remission. Enough to be significant, absolutely."

It's hardly encouraging that the efficacy rates for antidepressants have actually dropped over the past half century. But this may have less to do with how good these drugs are and more to do with changes in how we're measuring them: studies are getting better at differentiating between wishful thinking and statistically valid results. The under-representation of people of colour in clinical trials has resulted in meds that may not work as well in populations we know are already underserved. At the same time, changes to the way we define depression have included a whack of new people, which means drug trials suddenly contain more people with milder versions of the disorder, who we now know are way less likely to derive any real benefit from antidepressants. [20]

We're most aware of the people who aren't helped by psychiatric meds, rather than people who are, which could be exacerbating our confusion over what actually works. "We see and hear the untreated, acutely psychotic shoeless man screaming in the street, or our loved ones who have not yet responded to their medications. By contrast, the mental illnesses of our colleagues or friends who have remitted with treatment are invisible," says Benoit Mulsant, the clinician scientist with CAMH who specializes in "hard-to-treat" older populations.[21] He also notes that part of antidepressants' perceived inefficacy could be due to premature discontinuation: if you just go off your meds, or go off them prematurely, they aren't going to make you better. This makes sense. But if the best meds you have are so awful for so many and require such a long-term commitment that people in the grips of illness don't bother, then your meds kind of suck.

12

Good Noticing!

Combined with, and throughout, my variegated parade of drugs was cognitive behavioural therapy (CBT), which for me resembled more than anything an endless sadomasochistic Socratic logic exercise.

Pioneered by Aaron Beck in the 1960s,[1] it uses thoughts as levers to tame and defuse overpowering emotions: you record your emotions, the thought underpinning them, and the evidence supporting and refuting that thought in the hopes of getting a more balanced view of yourself in the world. It's supposed to make your brain more skeptical of its own bombardment of toxic convictions, carving out new, less harmful tracks of automatic thoughts and, hopefully, avoiding the vortex of inescapable despondent paralysis.

The evidence for CBT and a host of other psychotherapies in treating depression is pretty robust. Evidence-based psychotherapy has been found to enhance the effects of antidepressants[2] and lessen the likelihood of relapse.[3] Most people, when you ask them, prefer talk to pills. Most physicians either don't ask or don't care: stats indicate meds are used way more frequently, while psychotherapy use actually declined in the United States between 1996 and 2005.[4] I struggled for a bajillion years to do the "thought records" that are at the centre of CBT efficaciously. Long after I basically memorized the patronizing *Mind Over Mood* book and the conceptual structure of its written exercises, I couldn't make it work when I needed it most.⁵ All well and good to convince yourself of the fallacies of your convictions while you're mostly okay; not super helpful if you can't do it when shit gets real. Nonetheless, this method pulled me back from the ledge innumerable times. When I could make it work, it was great.

Mindfulness sounds flaky. The group classes are flakier. At my psychiatrist's urging I shelled out $600 for a course—not cool: this exhortation on his part was unhappily timed with a stint during which I was uninsured. The classes consisted of a series of early-evening two-hour sessions where a pair of practitioners, one a registered naturopath and the other an MD, walked us in a group through various thought exercises. The idea is to become hyper-aware—mindful!—of thoughts and emotions preoccupying you and, rather than becoming subsumed in them, putting a bit of perspective-enhancing distance between you and whatever the overpowering thought happens to be. I found their encouraging monologues aggravatingly saccharine but listening to other people voice their psychic hang-ups was illuminating. Realizing the similarities and constants between people's shit, as well as the striking differences, puts things in perspective in a helpful way. More importantly, despite my disdain, these methods actually kind of work.

I had to physically restrain myself every time one of the mindfulness course's facilitators chirped "Good noticing!" But noticing is, seriously, a helpful thing to be able to do. The mere act of acknowledging a potent recurring automatic assumption does sometimes help me curb what would otherwise precipitate a spiral of awfulness. At the very least, it cues you to notice when this shit crops up again and again. *Whoah, that's a bad feeling. What's that? Oh, it's self-recrimination. I'm thinking I should die because I've ruined everything. That's interesting. I had that same thought yesterday, too.* Six hundred dollars was an exorbitant amount of cash to spend on this, but teaching yourself to become aware of your own feelings, disentangling feelings from thoughts and separating both from your self is actually worthwhile. I still try to create distance between my self and my thoughts, with varying degrees of success. Good noticing!

TREATMENT METHOD MATTERS but its effectiveness depends on the person giving it to you. Despite knowing psychotherapy works and knowing which forms of psychotherapy work, most people don't get psychotherapy that's been proven to work in a way that's proven to work. Canada's psychotherapy landscape isn't quite the free-for-all it was three decades ago, but it's close.[6] In many provinces I could hang up a "psychotherapist" sign on my apartment door and start charging $400 an hour to talk to people about their problems. Healing crystals: $50 extra. Most regulatory bodies will specify the kind of degree you need or the school where you can get it. Almost none will tell you what methods are legit and which are crap, much less check up on you.[7] Credential confusion in psychotherapy presents yet another way to miss out on effective care. It's hard to know what you're looking for if you don't have a background in the field. As a result, a lot of people get therapy that isn't proven to work.

Even if the average therapy-seeking layperson knew what therapies have been proven to work for whatever ails them—and I'm willing to bet most don't—"they don't have a prayer of easily knowing whether a given therapist actually delivers," says Michael Schoenbaum, a senior advisor on the epidemiology and economics of mental health care at the National Institute of Mental Health.[8] One of his "formative experiences" in the field of mental health care happened at a meeting, watching the medical director of a major insurer bemoaning his inability to tell with any degree of certainty whether the therapists whose services he was reimbursing were actually any good at delivering therapy.

He is clearly still incredulous that, even in a field characterized by subjectivity and uncertainty, we aren't even acting on the information we have to make sure people are getting care (and organizations are paying for care) that actually works. We'd never accept a choose-your-own-adventure approach to dental abscesses but we're totally cool with that norm for the world's leading cause of disability.

Either way, it detracts somewhat from the relief of knowing your soul-destroying state of being is a disease outside your control if you're then told to think your way out of it. I had a bitch of a time getting the hang of CBT, especially in those low moments when I needed a cognitive-emotional lifeline the most. And sometimes, in the depths of a snotty crying jag in your psychiatrist's office, being told your thought patterns are "too outcome-focused" is not super helpful.

But I swear, I completed thought records and swallowed my meds religiously. Didn't skip doses when they became ruinously expensive or hoard them when overdose possibilities tantalized. I held my breath and willed them to start working. I knew I was running out of drugs to try. And I knew that, once that happened, we might have to turn to more drastic measures.

13

Zapping, Shocking and Burning Your Brain into Submission

When one drug after another failed to deliver desired results, at my psychiatrist's suggestion in the fall of 2018 we tried repetitive transcranial magnetic stimulation (rTMS)—a treatment still so experimental it wasn't covered by Ontario's public health system: my treatments, fifteen sessions' worth, were paid for through donations.

Like just about everything else we use or want to use or are considering using to treat depression, TMS began as a tool for something else. It zapped magnetic waves at different bits of your brain to measure brain activity and track what happened when those neurons contracted.

"That same magnetic field you could use to evaluate the brain could be harnessed to treat it," says Jeff Daskalakis, a director at Toronto's Temerty Centre for Therapeutic Brain Intervention at CAMH. He tells me as we walk through the Temerty Centre's beige-ish halls that buzzing your brain with magnetic waves every five or ten seconds will depolarize neurons—make brain cells pop on, then off. Keep doing it, and you might change something.[1]

The idea behind *repetitive* transcranial magnetic stimulation (rTMS—repeated zapping) is to do the same thing electroconvulsive therapy (ECT) does but in a lower-maintenance, less resource-intensive, less freaky way. ECT uses jolts of electricity to give your brain a hard reboot through a general seizure. The rTMS technique uses a magnetic field to give more specific parts of your brain a hard reboot and avoids the seizure altogether.

He explains that "to the brain, magnetic fields and electrical fields are indistinguishable. They both cause depolarization of neurons. But they do it in different ways." Electrical fields hit the cerebrospinal fluid like a stone in a pond—ripples everywhere, sending those electrical signals all over the brain. Magnetic fields, on the other hand, hit a targeted area and stop. "So when you stimulate an area that big"—he makes a circle with his thumb and forefinger—"it stays that big."

The plus for rTMS is that it's easier to perform and implement, and easier for people to access, accept and attempt. But studies so far indicate it isn't nearly as effective as ECT.[2] And the psychiatrist and ECT evangelist Charles Kellner, of New York's Mount Sinai, is dismissive of the suggestion that zapping someone with magnetic energy is a viable alternative for people who'd otherwise be candidates for electrically induced seizures.

"Patients can do whatever they want, but my opinion is that ECT is a serious treatment for a serious illness—rTMS is much more a faddish treatment for very mild depression. They are not comparable. They're not for the same population and they shouldn't be confused."[3]

Back in Toronto, Jeff Daskalakis is more diplomatic. He thinks the issue with ECT is twofold: first is stigma, the deep-seated fear that people hold toward it and that often is perpetuated by psychiatrists themselves; the second is ECT's limited availability—he figures the province of Ontario has the capacity to administer ECT to maybe 1 percent of the people with treatment-resistant depression who could benefit from it. "So rTMS is designed to bridge some of that gap to get people better. . . . [It] is potentially . . . a lot easier to tolerate. There's virtually no stigma behind it. And so the idea of having rTMS deployed widely across the province is very appealing."

(It didn't work for me, and my psychiatrist thinks it may have had some unpleasant cognitive side effects: I found myself unable to make the most basic decisions, the struggle to synthesize bits of information sending me into a panicky tailspin. But I tried it during an especially awful fall during which I could barely make it out of bed to go to my rTMS sessions, so perhaps that's why.)

A KINDER VERSION of the shock treatment that sidelined Jack Nicholson in *One Flew Over the Cuckoo's Nest* and elicited such horror in Janet Frame's mid-twentieth-century New Zealand madhouse prose remains, according to the data we have, one of the most effective treatments for cases of depression that defy treatment. Positive response rates immediately following a course of acute ECT, usually several sessions over a week or two, can top 75 percent.[4]

Whether you can maintain that remission or degree of improvement is another story altogether. "For people who have very severe depression, it's a very important option. And it's used far too little," Thomas Insel, the former National Institute of Mental Health director, tells me. When I first spoke with him by phone he was helming the country's public mental health epicentre but would shortly after leave for the world of mental health tech startups.

How does it work?

Science is still trying to figure that out. Some theories postulate that the seizures ECT induces somehow spark the creation of new, stronger, more active neurons. Thomas Insel compares it to manually rebooting your computer—"just hitting the reset button."[5] The single most effective treatment-resistant-depression treatment available is the neurological equivalent of a hard reboot—an IT specialist asking, "Well, have you tried switching it off and then on again?"

ECT has changed in the past half-century: pulses instead of a stream of electricity; general anaesthetic for the pain; muscle relaxant to keep you still; a styrofoam-like bite block so you don't chomp your tongue; a whole team to do the procedure, including an anaesthesiologist monitoring your heart rate, breathing and blood pressure.

You get electrodes on your scalp to measure your brain activity and bespoke voltage titrated to your brain's needs.[6] You turn on the electricity with a button and not, to my chagrin, the kind of fun-size switch I'd envision Dr. Frankenstein using to animate his creation.

The electrical stimulus is measured in millicoulombs, set at several times the minimum amount of energy it will take to induce a full seizure in a person. At the right dose, four to eight seconds of stimulus makes for twenty to sixty seconds of generalized seizure. The whole thing, start to finish, takes about eight minutes. Then you head to the recovery area and have some breakfast, because you haven't had anything to eat or drink in the eight or so hours prior to the procedure. Coffee can be good, apparently, especially if you have a post-seizure headache. The fine print is that you need these shocks to your brain repeatedly in order for them to work in the long term— the first round is maybe two or three a week, but "continuation" ECT in the months following the first round make you much more likely to stay well. And even then, your odds aren't amazing: 37 percent of the people in a 2016 study who got ten extra ECT treatments following their first acute round had relapsed within six months.[7] Just as worrying, for many, this treatment can mess with memory and cognition, although studies dispute how long the cognitive impairment lasts and how much of it is due to the depression itself. You'll probably be groggy for about twenty minutes after the procedure. You shouldn't drive a car for the next day or so. General haziness may stick around for a couple of weeks. Most people lose some memories—the most vulnerable ones seem to be discrete recollections formed in the weeks or months before treatment; a trip, perhaps, or a new acquaintance. Most people get most memories back within six months of their last round of ECT. But some are gone for good.

"It's not as big a concern as most people think," Charles Kellner assures me over the phone from New York. "There's no medical procedure without side effects, and some temporary recent memory loss is a side effect of ECT for many patients." He, for one, is tired of people's electroconvulsive (*do not* call it electroshock) therapy freak-outs. "The problem is that most people get their information from the internet. . . . Even Wikipedia, which many people consider reliable, the ECT page has been infiltrated by the Scientologists."

He also tells me that ECT is being refined all the time, its negative side effects whittled away. Ultra-brief pulses, for example, seem to minimize cognitive damage; ditto electrical pulses that target only one side of the head instead of both. But these somewhat gentler methods can also be less effective than the blunter versions.

Charles Kellner refused to talk about what percentage of people who get ECT lose memories they never get back, because "it will be misunderstood." He says, reasonably enough, that people forget things all the time and it's tough to separate what the ECT made you forget from what depression messed up in your memory from things you would have forgotten anyway. He thinks we should stop worrying about that, period.

"What you have to understand is you would never do ECT for a trivial reason. . . . If I were an oncologist instead of a psychiatrist and you came to me with a life-threatening cancer and I said to you, 'You need chemotherapy to save your life and the chemotherapy is going to cause you to lose your hair for six months' and you said to me, 'I'm not going to have my lifesaving treatment because I don't want to lose my hair,' it would be the same thing as a seriously depressed patient saying, 'I don't want to have ECT because I'm going to have a temporary, small amount of memory loss.' It's equally ludicrous."

Maybe this argument convinces some patients. Maybe being told you're being ridiculous and your concerns are silly and memories are no more valuable than hair, silly patient, can actually make you trust a treatment you were leery of before. Call me crazy, but memory loss worries me way more than hair loss. In my early forays into the mood disorder universe, the very prospect of ECT petrified me.

But it's easy to foreswear icky interventions a week into beginning treatment for this illness you just realized you had; much more difficult after a decade of debilitation. My ECT antipathy weakened with every new drug regime. Truly, I have enormous respect for the difficult decisions people make about their treatment.

My psychiatrist and I discussed it in passing but we shared the same concern: even if a workplace disability plan allowed me to take weeks or months off work, even if I were confident of a return to the office at some point in the future, how could I live in the interim, and how could I work with compromised cognitive capacity that could last months or years? I rely too much on work for my life's purpose and I have no brainpower to spare. It's not something I've ruled out. But it's something I'd think hard about beforehand.

I'm not the only one imbued with a deep-seated fear of medically administered brain electrocution. Rebranding electric cerebral jolts as less painful, more humane, less likely to cause grand mal seizures and proven to do wonders for people in the most catatonic states of depression has been only partially successful so far. Psychiatrists are fighting an uphill battle against decades of culturally ingrained, once-well-founded public horror of the procedure—so much that few public hospitals offer ECT.

WHAT ELSE IS out there? A hole in your head.

Your brain has no pain sensors, so you only need a local anaesthetic on your scalp before a surgeon makes a crescent-moon incision across the top, pulls back the tissue, drills a hole through either side of your skull and uses an insulated stylus, metal tip the size of the ball of a ballpoint pen, to burn two mirror-imaged spheres the size of sugar cubes in your brain tissue.

If you try everything and nothing works—not neurotransmitter reuptake inhibitors, monoamine oxidase inhibitors, mood stabilizers, anticonvulsants, antipsychotics, psychotherapy, repetitive transcranial magnetic stimulation or electroconvulsive therapy—you may qualify for what is called an anterior cingulotomy. The surgery, pioneered in the 1950s and '60s in the shadow of the lobotomy—the Nobel-winning procedure involving an ice pick through your eye socket to scramble your frontal lobe, frequently performed on men and women (mostly women) without anything resembling consent and with often devastating results—involves toasting two spheres of brain tissue about a centimetre in diameter.

I contacted Darin Dougherty—a psychiatrist at Massachusetts General, still the only hospital in the U.S. that performs these surgeries for mental illness—to find out more about the procedure. He was friendly and encouraging of my desire to learn more than the nothing I knew about brain surgery.

In the wake of what he calls "the frontal lobotomy debacle," the neurosurgery community was seeking a more precise way to slice into the brains of people with mental illness. Neurosurgeons didn't know where to start so they picked a spot at random. "The idea was to move from these big, indiscriminate lesions . . . to small, targeted, discriminate lesions," Darin Dougherty explains to me.[8] Apparently we still don't know how it works, though, or why we target the forward-facing inner fold of brain called the dorsal anterior cingulate cortex, or what that cortex does. But we do know it's part of the network that's involved in depression. "Remember this procedure was started in the '60s . . . and it just happened to be effective."

Similar surgeries were being pioneered at a few sites worldwide around the same time. But some guesses were less lucky. "In Germany they did things like excise part of your grey cortical matter on the brain surface. Yeah, they would just take cortex away, and that wasn't effective," he says. You had dozens of people in the mid-twentieth century who volunteered for an experimental craniotomy to treat their intractable depression only to be left with two holes in their heads, still mired in despondency. "Can you imagine?"

The trouble with these invasive procedures: you can't do a randomized control trial on a brain surgery procedure. The control would require a fake skull-drilling, brain-tissue-burning operation. All you can do is track what happens to the patients who get it. And the evidence so far shows that the cingulotomy that surgeons stuck with, that toasts two little spheres of your brain, still works better than almost anything for people for whom nothing else works.[9]

What's involved in an anterior cingulotomy? You come in to hospital. You get an MRI "so we know exactly where we're going." You get local anaesthetic lidocaine in your scalp, then a frame—the kind that looks like metal scaffolding and is used for people with vertebral fractures—screwed through the skin till it touches bone so as to keep your skull stable. Maybe also a benzo like midazolam for anxiety.

Then you get a high-res CAT scan and technicians overlay it on the MRI to give themselves a visual of where they want to go. "It's basically three-dimensional space geometry stuff." They bring you into the operating room and screw your metal-scaffolding frame to the bed so you can't move your head at all. The surgeon slices through your scalp, one incision spanning the desired locations of both holes, which will straddle either side of the front-ish part of your head. "If you drew horns on somebody, that's where they'd be coming out," is how Dougherty describes it to me. A precision drill bores a hole into your skull, through the protective swim-cap-like dura, until it just reaches (but doesn't pierce) your brain. "The drill is foolproof: it's designed to do this," he reassures me. "You don't want a 'oops, I pushed too hard.'"

And then?

"Well, then you've got a hole."

The surgeon takes the metal probe programmed with the exact coordinates of the spherical hole they want to burn in your brain. Based on the imaging, they push the probe down as far as indicated and lock it in place. Then, they turn the probe on. The probe itself is insulated except for the tip, which heats up to about 85, 90 degrees Celsius. The surgeon leaves it in place for about sixty seconds, and voila. Your lesion. Then you can take it out and do the other side. "And then you just sew them up and that's it."

See? Easy. It's about an hour, start to finish. You're home within forty-eight. You end up with mirrored balls burned into your brain.

I ask if they've ever tried just doing one side. "It'd be interesting to study," he muses. "The problem is, if you picked the wrong side and you need both, you'd have to do two brain surgeries instead of one. So we've never really explored it."

He doesn't do the surgery himself: he's a psychiatrist, not a surgeon. After the hole's bored in your skull but before your tissue's burned, he and his team are doing research with your informed consent to see what's going on neurocircuitry-wise when you perform different tasks.

While they're in there, they can measure single neurons firing during specific tasks. They take electrodes the size of a human hair and insert them in the same place they're going to burn later.

If you really want to zero in on a neuron, you've got to listen for it.

"You can hear the crackle of a neuron—we always have the volume up. That's the best way to identify it." (Yes, that crackle's basically the same sound as Rice Krispies cereal.) "That's when you know you've found a neuron—the noise the electron firing makes; that crackle that you hear is an action potential or a firing." That crackle means the neuron is sending a message—making a connection, issuing instructions. He and his colleagues are listening for changes in the crackling pattern and how your brain is responding, then they chart those noises. "The sound is converted to a curve that we can draw and then we do quantitative evaluation of that curve, measurements and math and that kind of stuff."

You go through computerized tasks, keyboard placed for ease of use while you lie on the operating table. They measure your attention, and what happens when they try to distract you; they'll get you to do gambling tasks and see how your brain responds when you make decisions, when you win or lose. Dougherty and his team are less interested in how you actually do at those tasks than what your brain is doing while you do them—how you make the decision. "Because some people are presented with a high risk and they're like, 'I'm going to bet low so I don't lose as much.' And some people are like, 'I'm betting high all the time.' . . . And then when you hear whether you've won or lost, people respond differently, and their brain responds differently. And so we're interested in what happens at different points all the way along."

You can't compare brain activity before and after the procedure, because the bits you've toasted are no longer doing anything.

About three-quarters of patients who undergo anterior cingulotomy improve within about six to twelve months. This is a good response rate, as far as depression treatments go. Dougherty says there's no evidence it impairs your cognitive functioning.

But you've still gotta keep taking your meds.

"The worst thing that can happen is a patient thinking, 'Oh, I've had the procedure; I don't need to take the medication anymore.'"

The relapse rate is "low, but not zero." About 10 to 20 percent of people who got better following treatment will lose either some or all of the improvement. (Going all the way back to square one is pretty rare, though.) If you relapse or don't respond in the first place, if you're in that unlucky 25 percent that doesn't get better after having bits of brain burned away, you can come back for a sub-caudate tractotomy—that's basically the same procedure in a different location, toward the lower portion of the brain.

("Yeah, I know there are a lot of -otomies out there," Dougherty says when I butcher all these terms yet again. "You're doing great." You can thank me when this comes up at your pub's next trivia night.)

As with almost every depression treatment right now, you don't know whether burning holes in your brain will alleviate your depression until you try it.

Mass General does two to six of these surgeries for depression a year. To be eligible you've got to have exhausted all other treatments, but Dougherty figures it's hugely underused. Many patients and doctors aren't aware it exists as an option. The sordid history of lobotomies doesn't help, though he assures me again that "this couldn't be more different than what was done in the past." Sure, I guess. Although knowing the area surgeons target was originally chosen at random—even though they're uber-precise about it now—is understandably freaky.

SO THE GOLD standard for depression treatment is a combination of psychotherapy—whose clinical effectiveness is seldom regulated—and a handful of meds that have gotten more tolerable but no more effective in the five decades since their antecedents were discovered by accident. When that doesn't work, the best fallback is a memory-thieving controlled cranial seizure that terrorized asylum patients seventy-odd years ago. The only once-popular treatments we've abandoned completely are insulin comas and the lobotomy. Even hyperthermia may be coming back into vogue.[10] Therapeutic saunas for everyone.

It's worrying, destabilizing, irrationally guilt-inducing to know you're running out of options for the thing ruining your life. On top of everything else I began to feel like a failure at treating my own depression. Was I taking these pills wrong in some way? Was I fundamentally metabolically flawed? It didn't help that there seemed so little method to the madness of drug selection: I was on lithium, despite my lack of mania, then off it, then back on four years later; we tried half a dozen different serotonin, norepinephrine, dopamine reuptake inhibitors. Antipsychotics; an anxiolytic; an anticonvulsant. So many cognitive behavioural therapy thought records I could do them in my sleep. I did thought records for thoughts I hadn't even had yet. I followed every directive, but despite myself lost hope in the prospect of a future free of paralytic despair.

We keep smacking up against the limitations of existing options. Our approach to the brain, the methodology underlying every existing approved treatment for depression, has all the sophistication of apes poking a *Space Odyssey* monolith. Which leaves us fumbling in the dark to comprehend a disease that's been on society's radar for centuries, and to get people in the grips of one of the single biggest public health burdens in the world into treatment that works.

14

Brainiacs

A pickled brain is cartoonishly brain-y. Like opening up someone's chest to find a pulsing fuchsia emoji heart. It feels sea-creature slippery to the touch. Firmer, less spongy than you'd expect for a bodily organ. Its bloodless putty-coloured maze of bulgy folds and creases is mesmerizing but it's clear the thing I'm holding is an inert facsimile of a human's multi-billion-celled control centre.

I don't know anything about science or medicine but if I was going to learn everything I could about this enemy, my illness, I knew I would have to go to the brainiac epicentres. So I went to the National Institute of Mental Health (NIMH) Human Brain Collection Core in Bethesda, Maryland—one of the most major brain banks out there—to hold, with gloved hands, pieces of pickled brain and answer a fundamental question: What can you learn from a dead brain?

The formalin solution reeks of sour yogurt and liquefied rubber. Don't splash it on your clothes or skin. Latex gloves are mandatory. It's getting rarer to pickle a brain this way: pickling degrades RNA, the ribonucleic acid you need to tease out epigenetic abnormalities. But formalin fixing is good for preserving cells' physical integrity, if you're into counting neurons' starfish-armed dendrites to get a sense of the organ's multitudinous connections. Flash-freezing a brain makes cell contents expand and burst through cell membranes the way forgetting your wine in the freezer makes it expand and burst through glass bottles. So sometimes you pickle and sometimes you freeze, depending what your plans are for this brain.

I discover the bulgy folds are gyri; the grey creases, sulci. While in your skull, your brain's encased in that protective vein-mottled swim cap of a dura, but you generally peel this off early in the dissection process.

Sliding gloved fingers over gyri, peering at brain bits on a wheeled table, I felt like a mad scientist. I also felt hungry: coronal slices look like cauliflower cut stemwise.

The most important parts of brain analysis are way less sexy-looking to the layperson. You break each pertinent flash-frozen section into tiny fragments—sometimes through pulverizing but often by sending it to precision labs that'll isolate individual cells. "If your question is how this particular cell expresses its particular genes, [pulverizing] is not the best method," Barbara Lipska warns me.[1] Trust her: as the Human Brain Collection Core director, she knows. A small (but taller than me) and quietly fierce woman with short hair she wears under a kerchief-bandana—she is in remission for brain cancer, an against-the-odds battle she won and whose scars she's written a book about—she ushers me through her lab and shows me how it's done. You extract miniscule pieces and ship them out in tiny vials to researchers around the world. You use a microtome—like the world's coldest, priciest, precisest prosciutto-slicer—to cut vanishingly thin translucent postage-stamp sections of brain you can then mount on a slide for staining or microscopy.

One of the toughest jobs at a brain bank is the ask. Way before tissue hits pre-cooled metal, before the brain enters the lab to be cryoprotected, frozen, dissected, analyzed, someone needs to phone grieving families in the hours immediately after their loved one has died and ask them to donate their next-of-kin's brain to science. I do a lot of awkward cold calls, but this one would be especially tough.

I find Jonathan Sirovatka in his tiny office, retro by comparison to the bank of computers in the adjoining lab used to search and sort thousands of brain samples by dozens of variables. He's introduced to me as an expert medical lab technician but he wields expertise in all parts of the brain acquisition process and has permutations of his script pinned to the wall and shelf space near the desk phone.

Here, every morning, he talks to medical examiners—the trained professionals who perform postmortems. They call him or he calls them and they tell him what they've got.

"The investigators read me the circumstances of death, the history of the person, and I make a snap judgment based upon what I hear, whether they'd be a good candidate. And most are not good candidates."[2]

You can't accept just any brain for research. Any number of maladies and medical mishaps can render brains unusable. They are so heterogeneous even within diagnoses, labs do their best to limit as many confounding factors as they can.

And of course, you want it fresh. Generally, you don't want a brain from someone who's been dead for seventy-two hours or more. But everyone decomposes differently.

"Let's say a person was shot in a Washington alley and was lying there for ten hours in the middle of the summer, a hundred degrees," Barbara Lipska tells me as we sit in her office down the hall from super-cooled ice chests full of brains. "Another person is shot in the same alley in the winter and fell into the snow headfirst. Which brain would be better for us to do molecular studies? Obviously, the second one."

Between 10 and 20 percent of the cases that Jonathan Sirovatka gets from medical examiners meet those standards. Then comes the hard part. About three-quarters of people shut him down a couple of paragraphs into his script. Right around the bit about asking for the organ underpinning their deceased loved one's consciousness.

"Most families are in shock: it's usually within twenty-four hours of the death," he says. "I get all ranges of reactions. Most people—I'd say 85, 90 percent—are polite. . . . But on occasion I get cursed at and yelled at and hung up on. 'How dare you be calling me at this time?' 'I'm grieving.' 'You need to have respect: I'm trying to lay my loved one to rest and you're asking for a piece of them? How dare you.'"

He isn't supposed to take a side. He can't cajole people into contributing to what could be life-altering research for people they'll never meet, who may not yet be born.

The next of kin has about two hours to decide. Sometimes less. If they say yes, they go through a recorded conversation confirming they're making the donation decision freely, knowing they get no direct benefit and that all identifying information will be kept confidential. Then Jonathan Sirovatka drives in a government vehicle to the medical examiner's office to transport the brain in a plastic bag inside an ice-laden insulated soft-sided cooler you'd use for a picnic or a six-pack. He's never been pulled over or been in an accident but brings a document authorizing him to transport organs across state lines, just in case. The brain's on NIMH's campus ready for dissection six hours after that initial call to the medical examiner's office. Sometimes sooner. And then you dissect.

The instruments look deceptively simple: a scalpel; a long-ish rectangular knife; tongs used primarily for handling the colder-than-ice tray that holds specimen sections. They slice the brain into forty-five meticulously cut pieces, dab them with a tissue to remove most of the blood and take a series of organ mugshots from front, back, side angles. They note any abnormalities before the pieces go into forty-five marker-labelled, bar-coded resealable plastic bags like cascading sizes of Ziplocs that are then secreted in huge high-tech chest freezers kept somewhere between -74 and -80 degrees Celsius.

It's a little traumatizing at first, Sirovatka says. He was sixteen the first time he walked into a brain dissection and the supervisor said, "Come on over, look at this. We have a beautiful brain here." There is such a thing as becoming blasé, he says. So straddling the emotional family side and the clinical dissection side helps him remember these masses of tissue were vital parts of human beings. Before he started making the donation-request phone calls, it was easier to forget the things he was dissecting had belonged to a person. "I was starting to have this disconnect. Now I'm speaking to the families. . . . I was speaking to a father about his son and I was telling him about what he would be asked in the medical questionnaire and he said, 'Yeah, we're happy to do that, but there's one thing you're not going to get from any of the medical records that I want you to know: he was extremely loved.'"

Melanie Bose needs no reminder of the personal side of brain donation: she convinced her dying dad to donate his.

She was visiting him in Arizona when the issue came up. He was going to refuse, partly on religious grounds. She dug up rabbinic teachings that it's justified to save another's life. "And I also said, 'Dad, you're going to be dead. You're not going to know about it.'" He laughed. He consented.[3]

Melanie Bose isn't tasked with convincing families to donate dead loved ones' brains. She's the one who does the detective work immediately afterward, calling relatives and friends and doctors to put together a detailed profile of a donor's life and mental health in the weeks, months, years before death. The quality of medical records is variable. Health care providers are starting to enter the late-twentieth century but most of what Melanie Bose gets is still handwritten and sloppily copied. Their level of illegibility sometimes necessitates a magnifying glass. And lack of detail can be especially annoying. Hallucinations? Visual or auditory? Inside the head, or outside? Who were the voices, what were they saying?

Things can get even more confusing if the individual's psychiatric history includes a stack of conflicting medical records. If you saw four different psychiatrists over the course of your life and got four different diagnoses, it's up to Melanie Bose and the psychiatrists she works with to figure out into which diagnostic category to place the brain. This is not a trivial thing: brain research relies on big cohorts—unipolar depression specimens versus bipolar depression specimens versus control specimens—whose clear-cut definitions bely their inherent fuzziness. These postmortem categorizations, retroactively assessing other people's assessments of your symptoms, show how arbitrary—and often speculative—our psychiatric classifications can be.

INDIVIDUAL HUMAN BRAINS are so wildly different from each other in so many ways—the relevance of which we're ages away from fully understanding—that it's still impossible to tell, looking at individual brains, which one had a mood disorder. Three brains of people diagnosed with the same disease will look completely different; three brains from people who've never experienced any mental illness will look completely different—how do you figure out what similarities the sick brains share that differentiate them from the well ones? In science, sample size matters: the people dedicating their waking hours to teasing out the phenotypic, neurobiological, epigenetic variations between different diagnostic categories of tissue rely on huge numbers to drown out the noise. You need analyses of hundreds or thousands of brains grouped by diagnosis and you need to use the sum of your findings to draw general conclusions. Doable, mostly. Or it would be, if the boundaries between categories weren't so fuzzy. "The groups are so ill-defined. . . . This is one of the problems: we don't know how to categorize these illnesses," Barbara Lipska, who so generously allowed me to explore her brain bank, bemoans. "And if you can't, then what is left?"

Since 2015, NIMH has been focusing more on symptoms and behaviour. That means zeroing in on hallucinations, suicidality, mania, for example, instead of whatever disease category a cluster of symptoms fits into. But it's tough to measure behavioural symptoms from dead brains.

The molecular biology she practises didn't even exist for brains until very recently: researchers mostly stuck to brains that were still alive so they could see what happened when you poked them or sliced apart big hunks of grey matter. Informed consent wasn't much of a thing back then, so you had living human experiments like Patient H.M., the now-infamous man who lost his memory when a celebrated neurosurgeon with a lackadaisical approach to ethics hacked a chunk out of his hippocampus.[4] And even then, it was tough to link action to consequence or do anything more than guess causation. The brain is too complicated.

We're only beginning to develop tools that allow us to inspect the brain at the level where biochemical differentiations are actually happening. RNA sequencing is one of them—it entails lining up long series of numbers and looking for patterns. Barbara Lipska and her team have been, among other things, sequencing RNA to see how the transcriptions of certain genes vary in different mental disorders.[5] It's "like a signature. It's like a code," she says. "It's breaking a code."

I went to see her fellow code-breaker Maree Webster, who heads a brain research laboratory at the Stanley Medical Research Institute just a few kilometres away from NIMH, in Kensington, Maryland. Originally from Australia, she used to work at NIMH with Barbara Lipska; now she runs her own show, a 680-brain lab that got so full she had to stop accepting new specimens.

In addition to conducting studies designed to replicate and verify what partners around the world are finding, Webster's team is also researching human neurodevelopment, tracking what proteins play key roles in infant maturation and comparing development in various groups of brains in the hopes of pinpointing the places where people with mental illnesses diverge from healthy controls.

It takes a lot of work, energy and money to keep hundreds of brains preserved indefinitely. Maree Webster's lab has fifty-five hulking chest freezers. She sighs. "So rent and the electricity alone cost a fortune."[6] I get to watch a technician using frozen cordite to slice a translucent tissue-thin sample of striatum, a cluster of neurons and critical component of motor and reward systems, fragile as a pressed butterfly wing or a scrap of skin peeling off a bad burn. Elsewhere in the lab the tiny tip of a minuscule tube is designed to dip hummingbird-like into a frozen tissue sample and emerge with microgram-sized fragments of brain.

Both Barbara Lipska's lab and Maree Webster's send tissue to researchers all over the world. Tissue packages from Webster's lab usually go by FedEx, in dry ice. The lab takes requests on the brain part and manner of preservation. A key condition: you have to send the results of your test back to her lab. Her staff have coded all the samples, and only they know which ones are control—specimens from people who had no mental illnesses—and which are not. This means Webster's brain bank has all the data from all the studies done with all the tissue of all the brains in the bank.

It's a full-time job just ensuring everything makes it through customs okay.

The striatum I get to watch being meticulously prosciutto-sliced is destined for Australia, about a two-day journey away. "Australia's really a pain because they're an island and they don't want any biological things going in and out," Maree Webster says. "Others are more worried about terrorism. I mean, Israel doesn't like dry ice going in." You can send brain tissue to picky countries, "but you have to go through a lot more rigmarole. They'll take it as long as you do all the right paperwork."

Barbara Lipska knows better than to believe any brain-science hype—the breathless headlines trumpeting a discovery that will revolutionize the field. Even if it's her own. "I've seen a lot of papers and studies that have been done very quickly and on very small numbers of subjects to just get published. . . . I call it scientific pollution." The replication everyone's after is nearly impossible to achieve and just as hard to define, especially in psychiatric studies: there are too many squishy variables at play.

For all this frustrating uncertainty, for all the limitations of baby steps you aren't even sure are in the right direction until a bunch of other people have taken those same steps, she seems to me remarkably zen. And quite certain: "I absolutely think [depression] is a disease of the brain based on neurobiological dysfunction. . . . On a neurobiological basis, something is not working."

. . .

THE NEXT BRAINS I seek out are in Canada. I head north of the border to Quebec, where Gustavo Turecki probes preserved brains—some flash-frozen and some pickled—in Montreal's Douglas Mental Health University Institute. He's focused on tracking strands of RNA and comparing differences between people who are sick and who are well; people who killed themselves who suffered childhood trauma and those who killed themselves and did not.

Gustavo Turecki acquired his own brain bank almost by happy accident: he wanted to work with colleagues who had a small collection of brains, maybe a dozen, from people who'd killed themselves, which they were planning to study for biochemical research. A commercial deal fell through, the colleagues who'd owned the brain bank went on to do other things—and he had a collection on his hands. Now his Montreal bank boasts about three thousand brains. Brains of people who've killed themselves, of people who've had Parkinson's or Alzheimer's, and of controls who had none of those.[7]

Turecki decided to zero in on suicide because it struck him as an urgent problem that remained maddeningly intractable. "Suicide is a fascinating issue, from a clinical point of view; not only because it's the only condition of psychiatry that is lethal . . . it's difficult to understand. And this is what we all try to prevent constantly, yet we have no objective means of doing so." He is sitting across from me in his office, a glass coffee table between us and the grassy campus quad in west Montreal outside the window. It's August and I can taste the warmth behind the air conditioning and in the dust motes at the window. As recently as the 1990s, he says, the mere suggestion there could be biological underpinnings to self-obliteration was anathema. "There were some people that were in shock to think you could study the biology of suicide. They were viscerally against it. . . . They [would say] it's reductionistic to think that suicide is something happening in the brain. They think that it's social. But the issue is that it's not one or the other. If you are very sad, to the point that you can't see any way out, so that you're so severely hopeless that everything in reality changes from how it was before, it is in your brain. . . . We don't know exactly where it's broken, but we know it's broken."

That brokenness is what Gustavo Turecki and his colleagues are looking for. They haven't found it yet. In many ways they don't really know what they're chasing or how to go about chasing it. But for now he's banking on epigenetics.

Futuristic gene editing notwithstanding, your DNA doesn't change: the blueprint you're born with is the blueprint you keep as you mature, age and die. What does change is the way that blueprint's interpreted. Your RNA acts as messenger, translator, photocopier. Different forms of RNA tell every cell in your body what to do and when to do it. Their instructions differ depending what's going on in your life. That's epigenetics. It means "on top of," or "above," genetics, and it's become an increasingly sexy field in our efforts to explain things not revealed by genetics alone.

Gustavo Turecki thinks the secret to suicidality lies in epigenetics. The way your RNA uses some instructions but not others, if it transcribes some genes too much or too little, is implicated in your mood disorder. That doesn't imply causation. But just being able to differentiate between the genetic interpretation of a depressed or suicidal person and the genetic interpretation of a healthy person would be huge.

How can inspecting a dead brain give you insights into what was going on when it was alive?

He characterizes the dead brain as more like a fossil fixed in time than a computer gone irretrievably dark, taking its hard drive and activity with it. "Dead," he says, "means, basically, the book was left open at one particular time, on one particular page. So you can read what was going on at that particular time when the person died."

In his lab I barge in on a young woman extracting RNA proteins from tiny snatches of different brains to compare their activity levels and check any changes in the transcription rate of particular genes. She introduces herself as Meghan. "The brain is flash-frozen, so we're hoping the proteins will still be active," she murmurs. If she's annoyed at my barging she doesn't show it, and seems happy to explain to me what she's doing. Meghan takes about twenty milligrams of brain tissue, puts it into a tiny tube and grinds it up until "it becomes a brain pulp, in a sense." Add some buffers, spin it down, boom: isolated protein at the bottom.

Turecki has seen pathophysiological distinctions at play, he says, in the brains of people who've been through childhood trauma. They have trouble regulating their emotions, dealing with what others would encounter as everyday adversity. And there's molecular evidence of that—fewer hippocampus receptors that detect levels of the stress hormone cortisol, which hampers what's supposed to be a negative feedback loop. So your fight-or-flight mode never switches off. "Which is, if you think about it, an adaptive mechanism for someone who was exposed to adversity.... The message these people get is that the environment is sort of unreliable. So they cannot sort of be quiet and rest and relax because they never know when they're going to get it.... [The mechanism] becomes maladaptive."

Brains are intensely, mind-meltingly complicated. To the point that we're only just beginning to comprehend their complexity, much less alter their functioning with precision. Even knowing the way trauma is expressed epigenetically has done little to change clinical practice. I am bad at delayed gratification and for all our huge advances the future of mental health care still seems decades down the road behind the doors of these labs, stacked frozen or placed pickled in high-tech freezers.

What is there for those of us unwilling or unable to wait?

15

A Dry Pharma Pipeline

Much to the chagrin of anyone stuck on a crazy medication merry-go-round, there's not much new in the pharma pipeline.

It's psychiatry's curse of serendipity: the major breakthroughs on which virtually all pharmacologic depression treatment is based were lucky flukes, stumbled upon while scientists were trying to fix something else.

Iproniazid didn't cure tuberculosis, as researchers of the early 1950s hoped it would. But doctors noticed that it did make depressed tubercular patients a lot happier. Eventually researchers figured out that iproniazid was disrupting the work of an enzymatic system called monoamine oxidase (remember that guy?), whose job normally involves breaking down neurotransmitters that could then spend more time bouncing around, available. This was around the same time physicians figured out that monoamine oxidase is present just about everywhere in the body, and inhibiting it in the brain meant inhibiting all the other stuff it's supposed to do. This is a recurring theme: pharmacological treatment of mental disorders has all the precision of surgery conducted with a chainsaw.

Imipramine, a couple of generations removed from a failed nineteenth-century textile dye, was used as an experimental treatment for psychotic patients in a Swiss clinic. It didn't fix anyone's psychosis. But it turned out to be a wicked antidepressant—one that launched a thousand copycat drugs and a $20 billion antidepressant industry.[1]

Decades of R&D followed, replicating the same couple of lucky breaks. But treatment development is running out of pixie dust. Steven Hyman attributes the half-century of less-than-innovative, extremely lucrative psychiatric pharmaceutical creation to "the false hope created by the first serendipitous discoveries."[2]

Steven Hyman heads the Harvard-MIT Broad Institute's Stanley Center for Psychiatric Research, is a former Harvard provost and former head of the National Institute of Mental Health. He was among the first people I talked to after embarking on this harebrained project. At first, he tells me by phone, everyone thought "these drugs would just be the beginning—that if you reverse-engineered what the drugs were doing, they would teach us about the mechanism of depression. And that kind of giddy hope wasn't really out of place in the 1950s."

Things didn't work out that way.

Instead, pharma companies spent decades developing "me-too" drugs—drugs with near-identical mechanisms of action as other drugs but with a small change allowing for a lucrative patent— based on those initial lucky breaks, using the original drugs' medical mechanisms as starting points to such a degree that initial animal tests for antidepressants were designed and evaluated based on whether the drug acted like existing antidepressants, not whether it actually quelled depressive symptoms. The drugs they created became more tolerable in terms of side effects and less dangerous in case of overdose, which is a plus when you're prescribing them to seriously serially suicidal patients like me. But they never got any better at doing what they were supposed to do: alleviate depression.[3]

If anything, the early flukes gave way to a skewed understanding of the disease itself: the idea that depression must be caused by some kind of neurotransmitter imbalance—wonky levels of the chemical messengers that regulate mood, among other things.

We know now it's far more complicated. And we're nowhere close to breakthroughs in terms of how depression actually works. While even cancer lets you take a biopsy and peer closely at a small slice of tumour, good luck hacking off a chunk of someone's brain. And even if you could, it wouldn't help. Whatever's messing with your brain isn't confined to one small fold of grey matter, a single snip of neurons. The screw-up involves a multifactorial maze within an organ we haven't begun to understand.

Drug R&D probably would have continued churning out near-identical versions of the same 1950s discoveries if buyers and regulators hadn't wised up and started requiring new psychiatric drugs to actually be demonstrably better than what was out there. Europe made the first move in 2013 , requiring all new drugs for treatment-resistant depression to perform not only better than placebos, but better than existing, pharmacologically similar drugs already on the market.[4] Why didn't this happen earlier? "Payers were dumb," Hyman says, then corrects himself. "That's not a nice thing to say. It's because marketing works. But the payers really should have known better." And once the rules changed, the party was over. "I think that really, in some ways, started the exit. . . . There are still a few companies who are in this business but most of them, even the ones that still have a reasonable number of projects . . . are actually investing much less money per project."[5]

Truth is, pharma companies don't know how to make new and more efficacious depression meds because nobody does. And it's hard to make money when you don't know how your secret ingredients work.

So, many are getting out of the biz and closing psychiatric R&D units altogether: Research and development is expensive and slow; the availability of animal subjects with brains similar to humans essentially nonexistent; the metrics of success increasingly slippery and tough to quantify. Any real, profit-making progress is a decade away. GlaxoSmithKline closed its neuroscience research facility in 2010, as did AstraZeneca; Novartis shuttered its brain research facility in 2011. "Progress based on neurotransmitters has become small and incremental," Mark Fishman, then president of the Novartis

Institutes of BioMedical Research, told *Nature* at the time.[6] Pfizer, Merck and Sanofi also retrenched their research and development in psychiatric drugs around the same time.[7]

Richard Friedman, the director of psychopharmacology at Weill Cornell Medicine in New York, recommended to me by Andrew Solomon, paints the same picture. "In the last couple of years [pharmaceutical companies] have really begun to shut down, if not totally shut down, their brain research science, because developing psychotropic drugs is extremely risky, expensive, unlikely to yield effective agents for all kinds of complicated reasons. So the drug companies play it safe. . . . It's not that it happened suddenly—it's a drip, drip, drip. But it's been going on for quite a while and they decided to cut their losses." After doing the same thing for so long with so few new insights or results, "developing a new compound with a new target is daunting."[8]

And, he adds, "Behavioural measurements, while they can be valid and reliable, to a lot of people are 'squishy.'" Uncertainty-averse people in the business of making money are not fans of measures that require someone to tell you about the kinds of deep-seated emotions and soul-destroying self-conceptions the patient has spent ages trying to suppress or hide or ignore.

Okay, but what do pharma companies themselves have to say about this neglected and unattractive field? I reached out to some of the biggest players to get their takes on why depression gets no love.

Lilly, maker of Prozac, the drug that's become synonymous with depression pharmacotherapy, as well as big-name newbies such as Cymbalta, declined my request to chat. "Thank you for reaching out to us. We're not able to grant an interview at this time, but I know there are many external resources on this subject. You can also visit Lilly.com for a timeline of discoveries if that's helpful," Lilly's spokesperson wrote in an email.[9]

Pfizer, maker of Effexor and Zoloft, the latter one of the most popular drugs in the United States as recently as 2013 and whose generic version I popped for years, did not want to be interviewed either. "That is not an area of focus for us now. Thanks for the offer, but we'll pass," a spokesman wrote back.[10]

Sanofi declined to speak with me when I asked, because "treatment of depression and suicide is not an area Sanofi concentrates [its] efforts."[11] Ditto Merck. "Depression is not an area that Merck currently has compounds in development, per our corporate pipeline chart. I would refer you to others in the field involved in this area of research."[12]

Allergan, which is one of the few major companies making new depression treatments, initially responded to an email request for an interview but then, when I followed up, did not get back to me.[13]

"If you are the CEO of a drug company and your job depends on your revenue and your profits," Steven Hyman points out, "it's pretty obvious the brain seems too hard, too risky. . . . I was trying to convince . . . some companies to stay involved with schizophrenia, and the head of discovery said, 'Look—this might help my successor's successor, but how will it help me?'"[14]

The pharmaceutical industry's commercial imperatives are not kind to depression drug research. Shareholders know that. "They look at the portfolio of the company," says Ken Kaitin, head of the Tufts Center for the Study of Drug Development, who I turned to for clarity in sorting out why there's so little new on the depression treatment horizon, "and if they see the company is focusing on antidepressants, they're going to say, 'Sell. I don't want this stock anymore, because I'm not interested in a company that's developing drugs that are not going to be big sellers.'"[15]

The smart pharma money right now is on cancer: cancer is way ahead and advancing faster; there are actual genes to target. Huge public support has been tremendously effective in raising money and awareness. And new cancer drugs can command a very high price.

The one thing depression drugs have going for them is market potential: there's a big unmet need, and a higher disease burden, overall, than for cancer. But need is not enough—the millions of people who will buy your novel new depression drug for years, if not decades, are not themselves adequate incentive for anyone to want to invest the time and money required to make that drug.

When it comes to drug research the deck is stacked against psychiatric conditions in general and depression in particular, Ken Kaitin says. To drive pharmaceutical R&D in a particular disease area you need scientific knowledge, an economic environment that makes for a strong business case, a market demand and a risk level that allows you a degree of confidence that your new compound is going to succeed, and depression drugs face a real challenge in all those areas. "Bottom line is, the competitive landscape, scientific knowledge and technical risks, all those negatives outweigh the positives of a positive market environment." And prospective psych drugs take longer to go through clinical testing than others—about nine years, on average, compared to five or six. That means added hassle and cost but it also shortens the amount of time you have exclusive dibs on the product. And that's assuming you get approval. Psych drugs fail at a higher rate than any other drug type out there, he says—their success rate is about half the industry average.

Richard Friedman argues it's time to rip up the existing model for depression drug development and start over. Instead of waiting for pharma companies to come up with something fun and new, he would like to see publicly subsidized researchers identify novel compounds and take those to corporations to turn them into marketable drugs. But not everyone is on board: Ken Kaitin is skeptical about getting government and other publicly funded bodies too deeply involved in what he sees as commercial drug development. He'd like to see multi-party partnerships whose aim is to devise new treatments for conditions where the public interest in breakthroughs outweighs the private-sector appetite for risk. There's a multi-party Alzheimer's Disease Neuroimaging Initiative in Japan, Australia and Brazil. And America's National Institutes of Health has started an accelerated medicines partnership targeting drugs to treat lupus, rheumatoid arthritis, diabetes and Alzheimer's.

None of this exists for depression.

"The emotional toll," Kaitin says, "of something like Alzheimer's disease or cancer, that drives a lot of passion. And it drives a lot of fear among people [which] they fall prey to. You don't see that in areas like depression.

"For lack of a better word, it's not sexy in the same way."

Fact-check: true. Depression is not sexy enough for the spotlight. A major reason we neglect depression—even more than we neglect other psychiatric illnesses—is because the most devastating disease in the world, in terms of total disease burden, lacks that certain je ne sais quoi.

Governments, at least so far, have not stepped in to match the cash lost by the private sector's exit. America's National Institute of Mental Health is losing its research capacity;[16] Canada's federal and provincial governments have made big promises about boosting funding for brain research but we're only beginning to see that cash materialize. Mental health research gets one-third the public funding cancer research gets, despite having, according to the World Health Organization, a higher burden of disease.[17] And even within organizations dedicated to brain research, depression is not a sought-after subject: only one of the thirty-two Canada Brain Research Fund projects awarded in 2014 went to a depression-related initiative—one focusing on the use of transcranial magnetic stimulation as a way to treat treatment-resistant depression.[18]

So cash flow is a major issue. For all the stigma-busting, mental health boosterism coming from political circles of late, it's empty rhetoric if it doesn't come with funding attached.

Anyone waiting for better depression drugs—and (have I mentioned?) there are millions—has a lengthy wait. The prospect of a breakthrough a decade down the road is galvanizing if you're a researcher or health-care practitioner dedicating your life to this stuff. But if you measure profit and growth in quarters rather than quarter-centuries, or if you wake up each morning wishing you hadn't, it's not terribly encouraging.

"We could be lucky," Steven Hyman says to me in a voice that suggests you shouldn't bank on luck. "But actually really novel, important treatments may be well more than a decade away. Which is heartbreaking. It's not hopeless, but it's hard."

Like, ten-years-without-fancy-new-meds hard.

16

Old Illness, New Tricks—
The Electrode in Your Brain

So the status quo sucks. We're dropping the ball when it comes to coming up with better ways to treat a pernicious condition. But there are some avenues of inquiry that could provide new tricks for tackling an old illness.

Helen Mayberg was drawn to psychiatry but not the psychology part, so she went into neurology, focusing on looking beyond the neurochemical models that have been our mainstay for decades, to map the brain circuits involved in depression, incorporating brain connections with imaging technologies that allow us to read the brain. She was drawn to depression, she tells me, because she felt neurology largely ignored it.

Mayberg talks, quietly but firmly, like someone at the forefront of her field because she is. In her work at Emory University and, since I spoke with her, in her new gig as founding director of the Center for Advanced Circuit Therapeutics at the Mount Sinai Health System in New York, she tries to pinpoint what brain activity abnormalities are present in depressed people and aren't there in people who aren't depressed, how those abnormalities change in people who get better with treatment, and what differentiates people who don't get better on those treatments from those who do. As technology evolves, researchers have gone from simply observing brain function to intervening in it—seeing what happens when you stimulate one part versus another in different circumstances in people with different pathologies.

Eventually, Helen Mayberg hopes, you'll be able to do a brain scan before starting someone on treatment and use it to decide what treatment will work best on that person.

"There are people who need therapy and should never go near a drug: it will not work. And, equally, there are people who need a drug and it doesn't matter how badly they want to do it without drugs, it's not going to work," she says. The present trial-and-error modality "is very demoralizing. . . . You have to give people what their brain needs, period."[1]

She thinks brain imaging and brain stimulation hold the key to better depression diagnosis, treatment and treatment selection. But "everyone has a bias. If you're a geneticist, you think genetics is the answer. If you're a chemist, you think chemistry is the answer. I'm a neurologist: I think the brain is going to be effective. But I set up my experiments to prove myself wrong."

Wonky circuitry's role in depression notwithstanding, the science of neuroimaging is not nearly as reliable as news coverage of sci-fi brain scans suggests. In a 2009 study researchers showed an Atlantic salmon a series of photographs of humans in various social situations. The salmon was asked to determine what emotion the person in the photo was experiencing. The salmon was dead. Their scan returned neural activation results anyway. The falsest of false positives. The researchers concluded that the likelihood of random noise giving you misleading results in a scan involving some 130,000 separate bits of information necessitates multiple comparison controls.[2] You've got to curb your neuroimaging enthusiasm, calculate the likelihood of noise and check to make sure the pretty colours you're looking at aren't just dead fish brainwaves.

Over the years, Helen Mayberg's work studying what's going on in the brains of profoundly depressed people led to new ideas about how to treat people who don't respond to anything out there. Enter deep brain stimulation (DBS), where you implant electrodes in someone's brain and a mini-pacemaker below their collarbone. It isn't FDA-approved for depression but is already used for Parkinson's and extreme cases of treatment-resistant epilepsy. Instead of burning spheres in your brain, as in a cingulotomy, Mayberg pioneered a method of implanting electrodes in your brain, attaching them to a battery-powered pulse generator, switching it on, and leaving it there, in the hopes that the ongoing electrical stimulus will right whatever's listing in your brain activity. It had great results and then it didn't and researchers are trying to figure out why.

DBS surgery begins in a fashion similar to cingulotomies: with an MRI. Local lidocaine to numb your scalp. Metal scaffolding frame affixed to your head, then to the bed once you're wheeled into the operating room, so your head, neck, skull are immobile. Another scan. A precision drill bores holes through your skull, but instead of the anterior cingulate cortex (that place where your horns, if you had them, would be), Mayberg's team threads a pair of tiny electrodes a bit lower down, into what's known as Brodmann area 25, which tends to be too hyperactive in depression.

The tiny electrodes are then connected via spiderweb-thin wires to a battery-operated implant—a pulse generator—that's inserted under your collarbone during a separate surgery.

Mayberg and her colleagues were surprised how quickly it worked on people for whom it was effective. One of her first patients, having had that node implanted and turned on the very first time in 2004, told Mayberg it felt like an Off switch for her depression. That patient was Deanna Cole-Benjamin, who spoke with me in a Kingston, Ontario, coffee shop one November morning a dozen years after she lay in an operating room, smelling and hearing the surgeons drilling holes through her skull.

"When they're drilling, it's noisy," a cross between a dentist's drill and something you'd use for home renovations. "You feel the vibrations and you smell it. Kind of like a burning smell, I guess."[3]

And then she overheard her brain.

At first she thought one of the many machines she'd been hooked up to was malfunctioning. But it was her brain activity expressed aurally.

"You hear the electricity in your brain, you hear the synapses. It just sounds like radio static, or a TV station that's not in tune. Like, 'chhhhh' the whole time. . . .

"So that was sort of cool."

Deanna was in a Toronto operating room, becoming the sixth person in the world to receive DBS for depression.

She'd spent most of the previous four years living in a Kingston, Ontario, psychiatric hospital in the grips of a depression that sucked her under out of the blue one summer. She came to that operating table borne by desperation: nothing else had worked. After years of trial and error and error and error, her doctor called up a colleague in Toronto who was trying out an invasive new depression treatment. Would his patient be a good candidate?

It sounded crazy, but if anything, the total foreignness of the procedure, the lack of any cultural association, positive or negative, actually made its imagining less scary. "We really felt like we were coming to the end of a road. . . . We just thought, if there's an option, we have to take it." So there she was, in the operating room, scalp anaesthetized, screws of a stereotactic metal scaffold pinning her head in place. She remembers a room full of people, the procedure so new it was spectacle. Surgeons sliced and peeled back a flap of skin, drilled burr holes through her skull and wove hair-thin flexible filaments, tips studded with tiny electrodes, into her brain tissue. They turned on the electrical stimulus, snaked the electrodes into a different location, turned on the stimulus again—to see how she'd respond with electrical jolts at different places. Kept asking her questions—Is it sunny outside?—to ensure her cognitive faculties remained intact while they tinkered inside her head. With the electrode in one particular position, Deanna remembers seeing Helen Mayberg's eyes—"Elizabeth Taylor eyes"—as though for the first time. And, all of a sudden, an optical assault of psychedelic colours—like going from Kansas to Oz. So vibrant she felt nauseous, needed sunglasses.

"It was really, truly, like a light switch went on. I processed colour that I hadn't processed at all in those four years."

The sensation disappeared when the electrode was moved or the current was switched off but it was a sign to her doctors that they'd found a sweet spot.

Then general anaesthetic for another surgery, this one putting a pulse generator beneath her clavicle and threading the twin wires wormed into her brain down inside the right side of her neck and connecting them to her new battery pack. In the Kingston coffee shop she lets me feel the ridged uneven bumps of skin on her right upper chest and on either side of the top of her head. Surgical souvenirs.

They didn't flip her switch right away: Deanna returned to the Toronto hotel where she was staying to recover, then went back to hospital to have the current turned on. Then back and forth for months to figure out what level of electricity worked best. First big shifts, to find a setting that made enough of a difference that Deanna was well enough to return home to Kingston; then "a little bit of fiddling" she'd drive into town for. "They literally just hold a remote control over the battery. . . . There's an On and an Off button and there's an Up and a Down button, and it's like a phone screen so you can see the voltage."

And, somehow, the numbness lifted.

For the first time in four years, she could hug her kids and feel it.

She returned to work, astonishing herself. "That was never even a goal." In some ways, the transition was weirder for her colleagues than it was for herself. "Not, 'She's a loose cannon; we can't trust her,' but, 'Let's not give her too much because we don't want to stress her out.' That took a period of time for people to feel confident that I was okay."

Deanna's had electrodes buzzing in her brain ever since. Lows like her grandmother's death a couple of years later were bad, but not nearly as catastrophic as she'd feared. She goes back under the knife every couple of years to get the pulse generator removed from her chest cavity and the battery replaced.

"It's a bit of a pain. But it works. . . . I don't want to go there ever again in my life."

The excitement over DBS's initial success was contagious enough to infect commercial medical device-makers, who went forward with clinical trials. The two trials—one by Medtronic, a maker of high-tech surgical, cardiovascular, gastrointestinal and neurological tools; the other by St. Jude Medical, maker of the now-ubiquitous mechanical late-1970s heart valves, among other things—both flopped. The Medtronic study was "discontinued owing to perceived futility" after failing to show significant improvement compared to sham treatment after sixteen weeks; St. Jude's was discontinued after an analysis predicted the probability of a successful outcome to be 17.2 percent, at most.[4]

St. Jude Medical declined my request for an interview. "Unfortunately we do not have FDA approval to offer DBS for depression. We conducted a trial years ago, but we do not have that indication and can't talk about it outside of a research context," a spokesperson wrote in an email, suggesting I speak with Helen Mayberg.[5] Medtronic declined too. Talking to me without FDA approval "would constitute off-label promotion," a spokesperson wrote in an email whose chain included a delicious forwarded note from another Medtronic comms person: "I normally don't support books . . . [ellipsis in original] passing this request if it's of interest. No clue who this person is."[6]

The studies' failures were a blow to Mayberg. Talking to her more than a year later, in early 2016, it still stung.

"My advice [to them] was, 'You don't know enough to proceed [with clinical trials yet].' They thought they did. . . . It's wildly disappointing to see something I know works not do well in the trial. . . . That's just maddening. How can it not be? You can only set examples by publishing your results, demonstrating that what you did worked, and hope that people follow suit. I'm not queen, okay."

What may have happened, she said, is that the researchers mistook a shift from the emotional flatlining of despondence to a fluctuating instability as a bad sign, when it may have been the mind shaking itself awake. Or the researchers picked the wrong patients in the first place. She suspects no one will want to pursue this kind of clinical trial again until they have a reliable biomarker with which to pick the right candidates. But none of this has dampened her faith in her method or her plans to pursue it. What she's left asking herself is whether it's ethical to provide a treatment that's been shown to work in individual cases but not in clinical trials; whether it's ethical to deny it to desperate people who've exhausted all other options.

She figures more than three hundred patients have gotten DBS for depression at three different brain sites. In most cases, over the long term, Mayberg says, it works—"It doesn't mean they can't have bad days or even depressions but they are no longer treatment resistant as they were prior."[7]

There's certainly demand for it, although most of the people banging down Helen Mayberg's door asking her to plant electrodes in their brains don't qualify for the procedure: they haven't failed all existing approved treatments yet. "I've had thousands of calls to my lab, and we take one in three hundred people. Because two hundred and ninety-nine out of three hundred don't meet that criteria. They haven't had ECT at all, they haven't had effective treatment, and they're calling to get brain surgery."

THERE'S MORE THAN one way to plant an electrode in your brain, and Darin Dougherty, the psychiatrist and director of neurotherapeutics at Massachusetts General Hospital, is chasing a more precise way to jolt your neurons into health. Affable and patient, this is the guy who walked me through all the -otomies when describing the way surgeons burn sugar-cube-sized spheres in your brain to treat your depression.

The electrode setups that have been tried so far for depression—Helen Mayberg's included—are "open loop" systems, where the electrodes are basically in "go" mode from day one. Dougherty is working on a "closed loop" system—a bit more complicated and more sophisticated, he suggests: you have a responsive electrode that's monitoring your brain activity and, when it senses any abnormality associated with the pathology it's there to treat, it switches on and buzzes until your brain activity is normal again, at which point it turns itself off.

So what suspicious neural activity could precipitate electrode-buzzing? Darin Dougherty's trying to figure that out. You can't measure any of this well without getting deep into brain tissue so he's using people with severe epilepsy as "patients of opportunity, because we can't just take somebody off the street and put electrodes in their brain."[8] So while epileptic inpatients sit in hospital with a slew of electrodes nestled in their brains measuring seizure activity, Dougherty and his team run them through other behavioural tests to see how they respond to various situations that give researchers a sense of how their emotional processing is doing. Some of the epilepsy patients Dougherty is studying have mental illnesses like depression; others don't. So he can compare the differences in neural activity for each task between the healthy and unhealthy groups.

Dougherty's research team got a $30 million grant from the Department of Defense to study the use of closed-loop deep brain stimulation on veterans with depression, post-traumatic stress disorder, traumatic brain injury and substance use. Maybe the coolest thing they've made so far is a little box they implant inside your brain that measures everything—all the neural activity you'd otherwise use a wardrobe-sized contraption to track. This is the thing that would notice something wrong and tell various nodes of the electrodes snaking between the gyri of your brain to turn on or off.

Like the National Institute of Mental Health and others fed up with the maddeningly inconsistent ways the disease we call depression manifests itself, Darin Dougherty is focusing his research on addressing underlying symptoms rather than a one-size-fits-all label of depression. He points out that a diagnosis of depression has to satisfy five of the nine DSM criteria, yet two people could have vastly different manifestations of the same disease, even if certain symptoms correlate—can you wake up in the morning? Do you want to die? "To assume their circuitry is identical is somewhat foolhardy and, in retrospect, could explain why open-loop deep brain stimulation wasn't effective. . . . So we're not even going there again. Been there, done that."

17

Old Illness, New Tricks—From Psychedelics to Smartphones

Gerard Sanacora speaks of his work with a fervour out of keeping with his measured academic diction, peppered as it is with qualifiers— "as far as we know"; "for the most part"; "this probably isn't the same in all brain regions." "In my mind it is probably the most exciting development, at least for mood disorders, in the past fifty years. I really do see it as a game changer. . . . It just opens up a whole new vista of treatments."[1]

"It" is ketamine. Otherwise known as Special K—a hallucinogenic street drug popular at raves. Up until recently its medical use was mostly as an anaesthetic. Now it appears to be pretty much the fastest-acting antidepressant ever. It's been shown to work on people who don't respond to anything else. It's also a dissociative hallucinogen prone to misuse, its antidepressant effects wear off rapidly and while we know repeated frequent use can badly damage your cognition (and worsen mood disorders) we don't know how or whether it can be clinically administered safely in multiple doses over a long period of time. Oh, and studies of its efficacy have so far involved teensy test-group sample sizes. Even if you combine them all they're pretty small. "We're just starting to scratch the surface," Sanacora says, sitting at a table in the unassuming office in New Haven, Connecticut, from which he heads Yale University's Depression Research Program.

Part of the electric joy underlying this scratching of the surface is that, for the first time, researchers could be coming up with a treatment that brings with it a better sense of how depression works on a neurochemical level.

But the more Sanacora and his colleagues find out, the more complicated everything gets. It isn't as simple as having too much or too little of one chemical or another. It's more likely a case of too much signal or flexibility in one area and too little in another; feedback loops gone awry.

He thinks depression is less about chemical surfeits and shortages and more about the brain's ability to adapt to its environment.

Every experience you ever have changes your brain's make-up: neurons fire, new connections are forming as you're reading these words. Neuroplasticity is the way your brain stores and retrieves new information and the way it changes to fit changing environments or circumstances. If your brain has trouble adapting, has trouble forming new connections or trimming extraneous ones, that's a problem.

If depression is in part a plasticity issue, and if ketamine can remedy that even temporarily, Sanacora hopes it'll be possible to capitalize on that window of optimized flexibility to teach the brain new coping mechanisms, through cognitive behavioural therapy or similar.

It's still early, early, early days.

There's a growing pool of evidence indicating that first shot of ketamine is effective. But the numbers of people involved in these studies get a lot smaller when it comes to longer-running studies examining the effects of multiple doses. In order for a drug to be approved for a specific use (as an antidepressant in this case) you usually need to follow thousands of people to ascertain not only whether it's effective at a given dose over a given time period, but whether it's safe and what the side effects are, and whether the safety and efficacy differ in different populations. You need lots of people and lots of time for that.

Thanks to human misuse and animal experiments we already know ketamine can wreck your brain if you take too much of it too often or for too long, and that there's a very fine line between the ideal therapeutic dose and a severely damaging one.

"What I see clinically that really worries me," Gerard Sanacora says, taking a moment to curb his enthusiasm, "is people who take it all the time. There's good evidence that people who abuse ketamine or use it on a regular basis do have cognitive impairments. There's evidence of structural abnormalities."

The Food and Drug administration approved ketamine for the treatment of depression in March 2019.[2] (As of this writing, it hasn't been approved by Health Canada but is being offered in some private clinics.) But probably tens of thousands of patients had already been prescribed ketamine off label before that. For example, at Yale, Sanacora had used it clinically, outside of research, for patients that were very well screened. And he felt that the risk-benefit ratio justified the use.

Just don't try it at home. "I would never recommend that. Period. Zippo."

Queasiness around giving people a month's worth of ketamine to take home and spray up their noses goes beyond the drug's potential to be misused and diverted, sold on the street. It can also be dangerous even if taken as directed. Even Sanacora's patients who get it clinically have to be closely supervised every time.

"It's relatively safe, but if you start treating thousands or tens of thousands of people, people are going to die."

Ketamine is exciting enough to be enticing some pharmaceutical companies to get back into the game despite depression's business-case turnoffs.

It's easy to be skeptical of corporate bromides on the importance of finding new and improved depression treatments, especially given the industry's failure to do so over the past half-century. But Husseini Manji, head of Janssen pharmaceutical company's Neuroscience Therapeutic Area, sounds genuinely jazzed about ketamine when I call him up.

"Depression is so disabling for so many people. And for many people, they don't get an adequate response to the existing treatment.

And even if they do, it often takes four to eight weeks [to take effect]."[3]

Manji is heading up Janssen's ketamine research. One of his studies took people with treatment-resistant depression, who'd been depressed for at least three continuous years and had gone through at least six antidepressants. Many had been failed by ECT, as well. Half got intravenous ketamine, half got an intravenous saline solution. The results were astonishing: within two hours, 60 percent of the ketamine patients began to respond; within a day, 70 percent did. That's a huge response for any illness. But even more so for depression, for which, as he pointed out, most treatments take at least six weeks to kick in, if you're lucky. "This was staggering," Manji said, his serious tone belying the excitement in his voice. The magic didn't last long: depression symptoms returned within a week. But it was something. "That got everyone very excited."

He and his colleagues focused on intranasal administration, the way you'd spray a decongestant up your nose. It's simpler and requires fewer personnel than intravenous use—you don't need people trained to administer an IV drip, for example—but it's also a more efficient delivery system than a pill, he says. Pills are better for controlled, consistent release of an active ingredient as it meanders through your digestive tract and into your bloodstream. With ketamine, Manji said, you want it into your brain ASAP. "There's actually a direct nose-to-brain connection, so we thought intranasal administration might do that."

They also switched to ketamine's molecular mirror image, the esketamine isomer, which is in theory more potent—you can get an adequate dose in very few drops. Industry observers say it's also arguably easier to patent something that's just a teensy bit different from what's been in use in various forms for decades: so instead of having a cheap molecule everyone can use, you have an expensive, patented one (patents are important; pharma companies are not in this biz to be nice).

Manji figures ketamine's mechanism of action is several steps downstream from what we've been doing all these years. It's more direct, he says, than inhibiting the sucking up of neurotransmitters like serotonin and dopamine into the neuron. So if we're taking a more biochemically direct route, he reasons, that could explain the relatively rapid effect and why ketamine has worked on people for whom more conventional treatments have failed.

Yes, ketamine will make you high, especially the first time you get it. "You feel that the room might not seem quite real, or you don't seem quite real. You might be floating or something like that." But he argues that their studies so far indicate you can use ketamine chronically, under close medical observation, at least in the medium term, without it damaging your cognition. "If anything, we see cognition improve, because depression itself is associated with impaired cognition."

It isn't yet clear how long you'll have to keep squirting esketamine up your nose or at what frequency before you achieve and maintain remission. Manji hopes that adding traditional antidepressants and psychotherapy after about four weeks of esketamine will let you gradually reduce the frequency of ketamine doses without losing their ameliorative effect. But here, again, we need more longer-term studies with more people to see how that goes.

One such Janssen study published in early 2018 found people who got esketamine in addition to their regular antidepressants (first twice-weekly, then weekly, then semi-weekly up-the-nose doses) had better depression scores, on average, than the people who got a placebo, and most of them stayed in relative remission eight weeks into the study.[4] Here, again, the sample size was relatively small (sixty-seven people total, which meant that just thirty-four got the intervention in the first phase) and I'd wonder how blinded your study is if the placebo is water with a bittering agent made to taste like esketamine, but which won't make you high. Surely you would notice pretty quickly. Either way, encouraging to the layperson. It'll be nice to see how they propose patients hang on to that lessening of shit symptoms.

Janssen also tested esketamine on suicidal inpatients, who either got ketamine plus "treatment as usual" (antidepressant and/or psychotherapy), or placebo plus treatment as usual and found that it had significant effects, on top of whatever else they were taking.

But, I asked Gerard Sanacora, as we walked down the stairs of his university building and out into New Haven sunshine, even if you can alleviate someone's pressing desire to die in the immediate term—which, don't get me wrong, would be awesome—would you be any more willing to release that person from an emergency department or a psych ward knowing the magic potion you'd just given them would wear off within days of their hospitalization? He agrees he'd be hesitant, too.

Husseini Manji of Janssen Pharma admits there's been inadequate attention paid to the public health crisis that is suicide and depression. "Because the field is so complex and so uncertain, most companies have decided to focus on things they feel more confident about. Which I think is very unfortunate because the unmet need of psychiatric disorders is so staggering. Once we get more confident then we can make headway. Then [R&D investment] will all come flooding back. The hope is that esketamine is part of that new era."

FOR SPECIAL K as an antidepressant, the high is a bug. For magic mushrooms as antidepressant, it's a feature.

The first tiny-scale studies into the use of psilocybin capsules— pills containing the active ingredient in magic mushrooms—are predicated in large part on the positive correlation between the patient's "mystical" experience and a reduction in depression symptoms. Here I have to be honest: medical mysticism is not my thing. But that's the magic behind using mushrooms to cure incurable depression, so here we go.

Darrick May wants to be a psychedelics-assisted therapist but so far he just gets to play one in pilot studies.

The Maryland-based Johns Hopkins University psychiatrist designed America's first trial examining the efficacy and safety of psilocybin to treat treatment-resistant depression (a similar, similarly small study had shown promising results in the UK the year before). Twenty-four people with severe depression who'd been failed by multiple treatments would be divided into two groups of twelve. Each would get two doses of psilocybin a week apart but one would go through the process ten weeks later. "This way everyone gets psilocybin."[5]

You can't have a double-blind (or single-blind, or any kind of blind) trial when everyone knows whether they've gotten high or not: the placebo effect's too obvious. There's no good sham treatment to use as a control, Darrick May tells me. So, staggering the groups is not the gold standard, but is better than nothing.

When I talked to him he was in the early recruiting stages for the study. He wouldn't tell me much about participant criteria—how many courses of depression treatment they had to have gone through with no results in order to qualify, for example—because he was afraid people would lie about their medical histories to get in. That's how popular the promise of free magic mushrooms and hours of quality time with trained professionals talking to you about your feelings can be: he got calls and emails from people in dire depressing straits across the country; he had to choose twenty-four. "It's kind of a disheartening exercise."

Darrick May doesn't yet know what magic mushrooms' mechanism of action is. He seemed enthused about the possibilities but also realistic from a clinical perspective. He says studies have shown reduction in subjects' depression symptoms "was positively correlated to how much of a mystical experience they had—that score on the mystical experience scale."

I ask, doesn't the degree of subjectivity almost guarantee a confirmation bias? People who like the idea of a mystical hippy-trippy experience will love taking psilocybin, will report a mystical experience, and get better after taking it. He admits they're also going to be the ones to volunteer for the trial. "People that seek out this treatment are very interested in trying it and probably have some positive associations and really believe that it can help them. . . . So that is a bias. But it would be unethical, or it would be impossible, to give it to someone who doesn't believe in it at all or thinks it's going to hurt them." There are plenty of people out there who already self-medicate with shrooms or acid or ayahuasca or whatever hallucinogen they prefer. And, he adds, there's a lot of discussion in the psychedelic research community as to what clinicians' role is in encouraging or quashing that: "Is it ethical to recommend a treatment that can be so psychologically impactful, both positive and negative?"

He does recommend a controlled environment. If you're going to do psychedelics, use drugs whose make-up has been molecularly confirmed in a health facility, and do them with a doctor, he recommends—not in a yurt in a forest.

There's a lot of getting-to-know-you time before your clinical shrooms trip, May says: the clinicians guide you through the process (yes, they are called "guides"), talk with you about your life, your hopes and dreams and what the experience will be like. On the day of, avoid a huge breakfast—messes with absorption—take a urine test and a baseline questionnaire and swallow the psilocybin capsule with a glass of water in a cozy room with a couch, meditation cushions, incandescent lights and the kind of ambience I'd expect in a yogi's home office.

"For the first half hour we usually have them look at some picture books, like nature or mandalas—we just want them to relax during that period." Then you lie down, put eyeshades and headphones on and spend six hours listening to a music playlist and having an "inner experience."

Some have bad trips, but with all the preparation and in that controlled environment, it's rare. Guides tell them to "meet and greet anything that comes up, and be curious about it. If something is scary, then ask, 'Why is this scaring me?' and if there's a monster there, look in the monster's eyes and say, 'What are you doing here? What can I learn from you?'"

Who should get this drug? "It's too early to say if anybody should be getting this drug. I mean, it has not been proven that it does work.

There's only been pilot studies," May says. Even he, for all his belief in the power of mystical experiences to attenuate depression over the long term, doesn't see pharmacies dispensing shrooms any time soon. He doesn't think patients should be given pill bottles of synthetic psilocybin capsules. The practice should be restricted to the way it's being provided in his study: in six-hour sessions in a comfy room under the auspices of a trained guide to take care of you. "There's too much potential for bad outcomes" otherwise.

PEOPLE LOVE THE IDEA of personalized treatment. Everyone wants to be a special snowflake.

That's what biomarkers could make possible: if researchers can find those telltale, testable tags in your biology that indicate without a shadow of a doubt whether you have a given disorder, and what treatment you're most likely to respond to, it would eliminate much of the fumbling guesswork that now characterizes depression treatment.

But even if efforts to determine who's most likely to respond to which treatments pan out, that's of little use if we don't have effective alternatives for the people found unlikely to respond to existing treatment options. Congratulations, Patient 8473! Blood analysis has determined you're less likely to respond to antidepressants. Stand by while we develop other treatments and ways to test whether they'll work on you. Your estimated wait time is . . . about ten years. Please stay on the line: your health is important to us.

Don't tell Madhukar Trivedi, on the cutting edge of this field at the University of Texas Southwestern's Center for Depression Research and Clinical Care, that biomarkers aren't worth chasing. The director gives reasons for hope even among our interventions' limitations.

"The crux of my work these days is to develop and validate biomarkers. So the short answer is yes, we definitely need to identify specific biomarkers for specific individual patients."[6] Instead of having a clinician walk you through a series of questions about your thoughts, feelings, mood and ability to accomplish day-to-day tasks to determine whether you have a mood disorder, you could have a blood test or a brain test or a cheek swab or a stool test that would hopefully, Trivedi says, then match the right treatment to the right patient.

He acknowledges we're a ways away from being able to do that with any degree of confidence. Is he optimistic? "Depends on the day of the week you ask me, and also my capacity to predict the future."

Trivedi argues fervently that, for people in the depths of depressive misery, accurate biomarkers could mean the difference between years of trying different treatment modalities and hitting on the right one in a matter of weeks. But, selfishly, as someone who's been through an assload of meds, years of psychotherapy, and rTMS, and who may face the prospect of ECT sometime in the future, if I had to choose between funding long-term research into biomarkers and research into better treatments, I'd choose the latter in a suicidal heartbeat.

It isn't either-or, he tells me. "We have to continue research to identify new treatments. . . . But there's a lot of work being done to identify new treatments." And with biomarkers, "at least we will be doing this in a more scientific, rigorous manner and not trial and error."

Biomarkers are alluring for pharmaceutical companies who've been turned off depression research because the failure rates are so high, the screening and progress measurement methods so fuzzy, because we don't really have a decent road map to develop treatments. Biomarkers, he hopes, could improve that road map, making testing more precise and maybe shedding a light on how the disorder works, luring drug makers back into the field. They could also, as Ken Kaitin, the director of the Tufts Center for the Study of Drug Development, points out to me, make those drugs more likely to get FDA approval.[7]

And then there's the algorithm approach. It skips the pesky need for scientific breakthroughs and focuses on the product we keep churning out for tech giants: our personal data. As in every walk of life today, people are pioneering ways to personalize your depression treatment by harnessing your personal information and that of thousands of others. There are companies that will take your responses to a clinically validated questionnaire and use them to determine what course of treatment is most likely to work for you. Others use more "passive" inputs such as your daily behaviour to assess the state of your mind.

The potential for data mining would seem to be even greater if your phone becomes your shrink, tracking your mental health (or its perception of your mental health) in real time. "We need to get away from this paradigm which is basically diagnose and treat: we want to predict and pre-empt," says Janssen's Husseini Manji. "Wouldn't it be fantastic if you could, you know, get an early warning sign that someone's depression is getting worse, or they're getting more suicidal?"

Silicon Valley has been betting on big data and the desire for a psychiatrist in your pocket. Google's health sciences arm, Verily, wooed National Institute of Mental Health head Thomas Insel to chase data-driven mental illness solutions. Then Insel left Verily to do similar work at a startup called Mindstrong.[8]

The idea behind these companies is to harness smartphones and the wealth of information they constantly collect—where you go, what you search, whom you text or message, whom you talk to, whose calls you ignore, what you say or type when communicating—to tackle mental illness. That would give you "a digital phenotype—a way of using digital information to get objective measures of behaviour," Insel told me back in 2015, when he was still at Verily. "You can use that data to predict downstream events, like onset of mania, onset of depression, maybe the onset of psychosis."[9] According to Mindstrong's website, its team used machine learning and closely studied research volunteers to develop "digital biomarkers" comprising swiping and tapping interactions with your touchscreen to assess your mental state.[10]

Mental health apps have proliferated, surpassing ten thousand.[11] Evidence supporting them has not kept pace. For one thing, there's a paucity of randomized controlled trials testing how well these apps work.[12] But the potential remains huge. So does the potential for harm: among other things, "nonevidence-based applications may distract patients and potentially cause them to delay seeking care," John Torous and Laura Weiss Roberts write in *JAMA Psychiatry*.

Here I have to ask: How do you use that data, and who uses it? What do you do with that information when you get it? Where do you store it, how do you keep it secure? Who has access to it—the patient? Clinicians? What inputs trigger what kind of response? If certain health states mean you're robbed of autonomy, committed to hospital, would you want your phone making that assessment, alerting the authorities, your insurance providers? What about your employer?

I don't know whether my phone would think I'm crazy, whether my patterns of email and Twitter use, my phone calls with sources and texts with friends, my typing, swiping and tapping patterns, spell out something pathological. But I can say unequivocally that I'd be leery of having all that data collated and if the disclosures I make or the conclusions my phone draws could result in a chain of notifications that'd lead to cops showing up at my door and ushering me into a crisis ward, I would think twice and would probably avoid doing so altogether. But that's just me.

THE STRANGER ON the street beseechingly yelling at you to "smile, sweetie!" isn't harassing you: he's just looking out for your mental health.

That's the idea behind treating depression with—wait for it—Botox.

The premise is seductively simple: Turn your frown upside-down. Or, if that fails, paralyze your frowny face muscles entirely. If you can't make a sad face, you won't be depressed.

The multinational pharma giant and Botox-maker Allergan is conducting clinical trials in the hopes of obtaining FDA approval of Botox's use for major depressive disorder. But Eric Finzi, the doctor, dermatologic surgeon and author of *The Face of Emotion: How Botox Affects Our Moods and Relationships,* has been injecting depressed patients with Botox, off-label, since 2003.

"Botox is a way of influencing your mind, your brain, without you having to do anything, because I am influencing negative facial expressions," he tells me by phone.[13]

It's not quite the same as the Botox injections associated with people wanting to be wrinkle-free: he injects the Botox into your corrugator muscles, the ones between your eyebrows that furrow when you frown.

Your facial expressions aren't simply the externalization of signals initiated by your emotional brain: they send signals right back, Finzi says, as part of a hard-wired animal feedback system. By short-circuiting part of that feedback loop, he says, you break the perpetuation of depression. "If you have sad thoughts, you will activate those muscles between your eyebrows. And if you activate those muscles between your eyebrows, your thoughts will get sadder. So it's a circuit. And what Botox does is it's sort of like putting a clip and cutting temporarily this neuronal circuit.... If you're not frowning, it sends the signal back to your brain continuously: 'Hello, you have not frowned in the last month. Life must be pretty good out there.'"[14]

Finzi figures he injects a few depressed people a week with Botox to alleviate their depression. They're referred to him by psychiatrists, psychologists, family doctors. Because it's off-label they're paying out of pocket, about $400 a pop. On most people it works for about three months, at which point they need a booster shot. He's less certain that partially paralyzing one of your facial muscles will also prevent a depressed person from killing herself. "I can't say that [suicidal people wouldn't commit suicide if they got Botox between their eyebrows]. I mean, that's quite a leap." But he said he had one patient whose suicidal thoughts went away a few days after getting Botox.

But, I ask, if preventing a person from frowning means she's no longer depressed, wouldn't getting a person to smile do the same? "There's no data" proving that, he says. But "I think it's a good idea for anybody depressed to be laughing and smiling more.... I will tell my depressed patients to smile more. But I have no idea whether it works or not. I don't know."

I'm not a scientist or a doctor and I don't know anything about Botox. But if you told me to smile more in order to stop wanting to kill myself, I'd be hard pressed not to punch you in the face.

SO WHICH, IF ANY of these—deep brain stimulation, ketamine, psilocybin, biomarkers, Botox, a smartphone psychiatrist—will prove to actually work for real people in the real world?

The process of evaluating any new treatment should be the same, Sarah Lisanby, who was wonderful about letting me call back and ask dumb questions, tells me in one of our several conversations on the phone from NIMH in Maryland: What is its mechanism of action—what is it doing, and how does it do that? What are its effects on the pathology you're targeting—what does it do to symptoms and how do we know that this is what's doing that, and not something else? This is a purposely high bar, she points out, one we've yet to meet for many existing antidepressants.[15]

"The field is scratching its head," she says, about why the deep brain stimulation trials based on Helen Mayberg's work failed. But she suspects it may be an issue of network precision—not just where the electrodes go but what the spots they stimulate are connected to; not just location but tuning. Ten pulses per second? A hundred? That's part of what Darin Dougherty's trial at Massachusetts General Hospital is seeking to answer. "The brain is a complex distributed network, a complex system, and we shouldn't be surprised that initial attempts were met with limited success, because we need to refine them. We need to be smarter. This is a bad analogy, but we've all had the experience where we're dealing with a GPS system and the GPS isn't working and it's telling us to take an exit which is the wrong exit. And we need to give the surgeons a better GPS, so they know which of these nearby highways and exits to target."

This all sounds fanciful and far away to someone wrestling with bullshit depression right this second. But Sarah Lisanby's enthusiasm is catching. Like when it comes to smart wires that snake their own way through your brain. Existing wires are rigid. When you stick them into the brain it's easy to poke through blood vessels, damage tissue. Researchers are working on smart, flexible polymers that can be "snaked around blood vessels, so they can clear the tissue non-destructively," she says to me. "You'd like to have electrodes that can insert themselves and navigate around the brain structures. It's almost like science fiction, right? But it's science fact."

PART III

A KICK IN
THE TEETH

18

Stigma and Related Bullshit

I am so beyond tired of the word "stigma." Perhaps it once had reso-
nance. Maybe its utterance once conjured a concrete, clearly delin-
eated concept. But repetition has rendered it meaningless, the way
a surfeit of swearing robs cuss words of their sting. "Stigma" came
up in every interview I did for this book—with clinicians, with
researchers, with people grappling with depression and suicide and
with their family members. But its ubiquity in discourse lets us elide
the agonizing crappiness it describes.

So let's be really, really clear about what persistent stigma means
for people with severe mental illness.

> You're faking it.
> You're delusional.
> You're weak.
> You're untrustworthy.
> You're selfish.
> You're self-pitying.
> You're unstable.
> You're dangerous.
> You can't make your own decisions.
> You're dumb.

Your contributions are less worthy, more easily discounted.

You're a liability—personally and professionally and socially.

You aren't friend or lover or colleague or employee material.

You make other people uncomfortable to the point they actively
avoid you.

You're less loveable.

You're less deserving of effective, accessible treatment than
people with other illnesses.

You aren't worth the time or resources it would take to find out
more about what's wrong with you.

People would rather not deal with you or your problem.

That's stigma. It's gross and profoundly damaging.

POOR STACEY WAS just doing her job when she phoned, a representative of an employer's insurer quizzing an employee about a
sudden protracted absence from work. But instead of a malingerer
caught in the middle of a bedridden movie marathon, she got me:
crazy lady pacing her curtained-off corner of the short-stay psych
ward, shiftily clutching the cell phone she wasn't supposed to be
using. By then I'd been there more than a week—a lifetime by that
ward's standards. I knew I wasn't being set free and was about to be
sent upstairs at any moment. I was a jumpy motherfucker.

"Hi, Anna? We were just wondering about your absence from
work. . . ."

"Uh, yeah. I'm in hospital. . . ."

"Right. Can you tell me why?"

"I tried to kill myself."

It was the first time I'd uttered those words—vertiginously
terrifying and emboldening all at once. I freaked myself out almost
as much as I freaked out Stacey.

"Oh." Long pause. "Yes, I think we would cover that."

I realized later how lucky I was to have gotten short-term disability coverage, about seven-tenths of my salary, during three sick leaves at two different employers: two in the ICU and psych wards after suicide attempts, one when taking sick days on short notice threatened my continued employment and prompted a strenuously recommended three-week leave of absence.

I swear, depression doesn't make me fuck up assignments. I can write stories and break news and still achieve, some days, that immersive euphoric high in pursuit of a story, can lose myself in interviews about neonatal abstinence syndrome or opioid misuse or the Higgs boson. There are bad days and worse weeks—I almost missed a press conference about a fatal shooting because I was having a minor breakdown in a bathroom stall; I spent a panicked drowning week chasing breaking news on a caved-in mall even as I struggled to focus on anything but oblivion. I spent weeks going to work in a zombie-like state. But it was the periods between purpose-giving stories, when I went home and couldn't go to bed and couldn't wake up, couldn't get dressed, couldn't leave the apartment, that fucked me over. Again and again and again. I struggled to explain inexplicable absences: How do you say, "I missed work because I was flattened by self-loathing and I didn't tell you enough hours in advance because I was flattened by self-loathing" without sounding like a nutbar or a liar or irritatingly self-pitying? I gnawed my pen to avoid crying in a meeting with two managers wondering aloud why the person who worked like a fiend was showing up at eleven o'clock. When one of them implored across his desk, "Give us something to work with here," I caved and told him the truth and immediately wished I hadn't. In another meeting a year later—different manager, same reason—my self-control failed and I wept so profusely I embarrassed us both. How could anyone ever hope for a normal professional relationship after that? How do you make that anything other than a professional sucker punch?

I don't know if it's possible to convince myself, much less another person, that I'm not a workplace liability. I do know that every time I've told someone about my mood disorder I've come to regret it.

(So it's maybe weird, then, that I'm writing this book. And I'd be lying if I said I don't worry this mass disclosure will be something I regret. But sometimes some things feel too important not to do.)

We talk a big game about talking. Online hashtag culture creates a cult of confessionals. There's #sicknotweak (i.e., mental illness is a sickness, not a weakness). In Canada, a corporate-sponsored campaign called "Bell Let's Talk" spawns an annual flood of personal mental illness disclosures.[1] Various celebrities, from British princes on down, are big on awareness campaigns. In the face of our fetishization of openness, Toronto's Centre for Addiction and Mental Health psychologist Donna Ferguson suggests people pause before disclosing a mental illness, even to those closest to them. I interviewed her for a Global News online story. "You really want to know what the relationships are like . . . and how supportive people are," she says. "You never want [someone with mental illness] to tell people and feel ashamed or criticized or ostracized." When it comes to the workplace, she's unequivocal. "I honestly don't think it's employers' business. If you're off on a medical leave, you're off on a medical leave. Or if you're at work still, and things are not going well, some people feel comfortable saying to their direct supervisor, 'I'm having some symptoms.' And I think if you don't, don't. You don't have to. You're not obligated. . . . It's personal. It's confidential."[2]

Openness is key. Talking is everything. But there are days I want to shout her words from the rooftops.

In fact, know that by law in many jurisdictions your boss isn't even allowed to ask. But it's one thing to know that; it's another to feel pressured to disclose only to kick yourself for it afterward. I've found myself struggling to make my mood disorder sound sufficiently serious to warrant whatever weird absences or lack of drive I'm asked to explain while simultaneously downplaying any impression of unstable lunacy. Failing at both.

. . .

IN CHASING THIS BOOK I talked to people who'd experienced—directly and personally—the brunt of depression and suicide from all their myriad shit-ass angles. They trusted me with their most personal stories and in some cases I promised not to fully identify them, because being known as someone wrestling with depression can still shaft you in innumerable ways. And that's bullshit.

I talked to Mary in a bustling dark café-bar on Toronto's Danforth Avenue.

MARY

Honesty cost Mary dearly. It obliterated financial security in the event of death, disease or injury: any protracted absence from work will throw her and her teenage daughter into financial peril. Mary doesn't smoke or skydive or do drugs; her health and blood pressure are better than average. But she has depression and she told her employer's insurer the truth when asked. And now there's a hard cap on the amount of life insurance she can get. She's ineligible for any short-term or long-term disability payments, no matter the reason.

"I could break my ankle walking out of here and I wouldn't be covered. I could get cancer. I could get influenza. I could get all kinds of things but I get no coverage. Because I have depression. And that was the sole reason. There is no question that is the only reason I got refused."[3] At one job after another in both the public and private sector, Mary hesitates over the paperwork query asking whether she has depression. "I've struggled, really, with the thought of, 'Jeez, do I really write that down?' [But] I can't bear the thought of not being honest. And if they find out you haven't been honest they can void all of your coverage. And because I'm a single parent, I need some of it."

The purpose of life insurance is peace of mind so the denial of coverage because you're crazy is its opposite. Knowing you can't afford to take time to heal if you need it makes for a state of perpetual insecurity.

So I sought out some of the voices representing Canada's insurers (US giant Kaiser Permanente declined my request) and they emphasized that every case is unique. But the representatives I spoke with said it's unusual for someone to be denied all coverage, for anything, because of one condition.

Insurance companies are not charities. They're in the business of shielding themselves from financial risk. Life, health, disability or income-loss coverage can be denied if the potential cost is seen as being too high.

And often mental illness is too big a risk to stomach.

Insurers call it anti-selection—"a policy taken with the intent to benefit from it to the detriment of the insurer," as Claude Di Stasio, former vice-president of Quebec affairs and holder of the mental health file at the Canadian Life and Health Insurers Association, puts it. Classic example: you buy home insurance, then set the place on fire. But what about when the harm you do is to yourself? Let's say you apply for health or life insurance and you get it—either you've never been diagnosed with depression or you tell them about your diagnosis and they're cool with it. Don't even think about killing yourself for the next two years: your beneficiaries will get zero dollars. Insurers worry that people kill themselves as a ruse to bilk their carrier and get money for their family. (This is all, incidentally, a great way to ensure people never talk about the illness eating them up inside.)

"We're trying to be clean and not discriminate, but we don't want mental health people benefiting from claims they should not to the detriment of other people," Di Stasio says.[4]

Trying to die or harming yourself without dying is also financially unwise. Many policies exclude self-inflicted injuries, so if you need income replacement or care that isn't covered by the public system, you're out of luck. If you want to try to get it covered, you'd have to prove not only that the self-inflicted injury is the product of mental illness but that there wasn't really intent—that you didn't know what you were doing.

Karen Cutler, the chief underwriter at Manulife, Canada's multinational insurance company, tells me by phone that the company offers coverage to the vast majority of people who are mired in or have gone through depression. They're looking for signs that you're coping and stable—for upwards of two years, ideally—sussing this out through phone interviews, cover letters, questionnaires. "It's no different than if we're looking at someone with diabetes or high blood pressure. How much time has passed, are you taking your medication, are you controlling your symptoms?"[5] Every plan and every situation is unique. As I write these words I am eyeing the little pill bottles paid for (thank the chronic illness gods) by my employer's insurer. But if you have a history of being prescribed antidepressants, Cutler says, chances are you won't get coverage for those antidepressants. If you have a history of missing work, changing jobs, or needing time off work as a result of your depression, you probably won't get disability coverage or, if you do, it will be limited.

"And that's just common sense. From a business perspective, it makes sense," Cutler says. Being hospitalized for depression, even if it was multiple years ago, won't count in your favour. But, she adds, "when we underwrite people we underwrite with the lens of, you know, 'There but for the grace of God go I.' Our goal is to try to offer coverage, not to try to find reasons not to offer coverage."

DEANNA

Deanna Cole-Benjamin, who'd shared her story with me in the Kingston café, recounted how her suicidal ideation and her psychiatric hospitalization jeopardized not only her own health insurance, but her kids'—even after she received treatment that pushed her years-long grapple with depression into remission. "I was 'too high-risk.' They just said, 'If we are not going to insure you, we cannot insure anyone in your family.'"[6] She might have been tempted not to disclose her mental illness, Deanna says. But her employer already knew, because her crippling disorder rendered her unable to work for years, long after short- and long-term disability payments expired. She lost all her benefits and when she reapplied, her prior illness was already known.

That refusal played a role in prompting Deanna to seek work elsewhere. "It's terrible. And you're just contributing to that whole stigma: you don't want to talk to your friend because you don't know who your friend knows who might say something to somebody. That's not right."

MARY

Insurers aside, Mary's gotten better at assessing how someone in her personal or professional life will respond to her disclosure. She's had to. "There are always some people where, you know, 'Maybe I'm not going to share this particular aspect of my existence with you,'" she said. "You pick up certain vibes around people" in how they react to difference and craziness in others—in the news, on the street, in the office. Even people who think they can deal with it, who say the right words, sometimes freak out just a bit." I've had that happen. Friends, employers who make empathic noises, who convince me and themselves that they're cool with crazy lady, suddenly ghost on me, or turn wary. "They don't know how it manifests and they don't know what they're going to do. And I think that's the more difficult piece. . . . Like, 'Are you going to turn into a serial killer?'"

Mary's had depression used against her by romantic partners, "with the suggestion that 'well, you're weak. You're the weak one, here. You're crazy. You're the one that's the problem. . . . It's because you're like this that everything is wrong.' Which your brain is also telling you."

She's had co-workers who say she's just too sensitive to handle the challenges and setbacks of everyday life. "That you don't have the gumption for whatever's going on. You can't stand up for the tough fights. . . . I can hear one particular voice, and it's twenty years ago. And it's such an affront." The worst is the way comments like these reinforce your own self-loathing. "Depression is extremely isolating. And it's self-isolating. Your brain starts to tell you nobody will understand."

Then there's the flip side. People still approach Mary for advice or just to talk to someone who knows what it's like. "They want recognition that, you know, they're in the same boat. It's really an important touchstone to know 'You understand my situation. I know you can't solve it, but you understand it.' They may not have anyone else who does."

In her decades wrestling with depression, Mary amassed "an exceptional support network. I have more than a few people who are totally open to being there if I need it." But she's never tested that openness. She says she's paralytically afraid of being seen as weak, afraid they will think differently of her.

THE FEAR OF REJECTION, the sense that your very presence damages those you care about most, propagates emotional isolation. And the loneliness makes you crazy. You don't notice till someone mentions your vice-like bear hugs. Then you realize you've been sending meaningless weightless messages to random people in the hopes of striking up an escapist exchange about nothing. You've been atomizing human contact: tightly interwoven fingers in clasped hands; the feeling of leaning sideways against someone on a couch. You start weirdly wishing for time spent with dogs and babies—their social expectations are simpler, it seems; their methods of communicating affection more straightforward. How dumb is it that I, so priding myself on my independence and so prizing my solitude, can so graspingly need someone to talk to?

When I was a kid our family had a dog named Charlie. Gorgeous chocolate Lab. Shameless droopy begging eyes. Extreme affection. Unbelievable stupidity. He made a point of devouring the grossest things he'd find on walks—decomposing fauna, mostly; and seaweed, for some reason. He'd expel it hours later, one way or another, like clockwork. And on our next walk he'd do the exact same thing. Whatever synaptic connections are supposed to be formed to create memories and then retrieve them to inform future decision-making, that wasn't happening.

Same thing happens to me when it comes to discussing pathological misery. I try it. It's horrible. I vow never to do it again. Time passes. And inevitably the desire to vent is so great, the prospect of some measure of comfort so alluring, that sandy dead crab so tasty, I spill. I break the brittle shell holding everything together.

It's not supposed to work that way. People say, "Tell me if I can help with anything"; "You know you can call me any time, right?" And don't get me wrong: there are times I would reach out and feel truly heard, feel like I was grasping something solid for the first time in forever. And, believe me, I understand how soul-crushing it is to deal with severe, chronic illness in someone close to you. But just as many impulsive confessions I regretted. Usually because they led to unwanted consequences—a loss of liberty or the initiation of an intervention I wasn't seeking, or a sudden social or professional distancing, the way you'd shrink from someone snuffling on a bus. But also because in my most selfish moments I didn't consider what the confession that brought me relief would do to the person on the receiving end. Even if they didn't shun me or call the cops, I caused them distress and made them feel obliged to fix something that wasn't theirs to fix. (My psychiatrist would tell me to chill, that helping someone at an excruciatingly shitty point in their life can itself feel empowering, can be "egosyntonic"—reinforcing the person you want to be. But my god I quail at the thought of burdening people with my misery. Maybe I shouldn't.)

People bemoan the paucity of people coming forward about their mental illness. But have you ever tried talking frankly with a friend, colleague, relative about your endless despondency, your pit of despair, your incessant desire for oblivion? The disincentive from talking to anyone but your psychiatrist about your mental state is enormous. I'm the first to admit I isolated myself preventatively. Because fuck if that wasn't a trillion times better than having people ghost on me—grow irritable or terse or silent in conversation; leave calls, texts, emails unanswered.

In fairness, much or all of this was probably in my head. That's how a negative cognitive bias works. But imagined or not, it is misery-making.

The result is threefold:

> You learn to interact with others as little as possible.
> When you do interact, you disclose as little as possible about your affective state.
> When you do disclose, whether out of trust or obligation, you learn to couch despair in something safer—pithy pissiness works well.

So the ice stays unbroken. Thickens, if anything. And the conviction you're actually horrible for other people makes an even greater case for self-annihilation.

I have more photos shot from inside my apartment than anyone living alone in a five-hundred-square-foot space with one window should ever have. I talk to the radio and to podcasts. Apologize when dropping or knocking over household objects. Chide contumacious hard drives, internet connections, appliances. A crazy cat lady with no cats. This makes being in places with other people even worse because I can't shake the habit of talking to myself, my computer, my phone. I laugh it off when colleagues murmur, "Anna, sitting beside you is so entertaining," inwardly thinking *I shouldn't be around human beings*.

Being a shut-in also gives you convenient access to a demarcated pacing area. If I don't develop a cardiovascular illness brought on by a fatally sedentary lifestyle it'll be thanks to pacing. That, and hand-wringing—both major medals in the Neurotic Olympics.

. . .

IT'S STRIKING HOW POWERFUL a factor shame was—is—in worsening my worst moments, making pits of despair inescapable traps. If self-loathing or insides made of lead kept me immoveable in bed in the morning, shame kept me from reaching for my phone when I reached consciousness to email my boss and call in sick, shame made me dread my workplace. Shame kept me at work later to make up for these absences, which further messed up my nights and doomed my mornings. Shame and fear of appearing a slacker stopped me from telling my boss I would have to dash out to an afternoon medical appointment, so I was late or cancelled altogether (in my defence, the latter only ever happened once). Shame stopped me from bugging my doctor or my friends when I was at home steeped in misery. Shame, horror at the prospect of ever having to face the world again, let alone having to face it and to face up to myself again and again for what could be the better part of a century, propelled me closer to death than anything else ever did.

Pro-tip: Don't sob on things you can't machine wash. Learn how to fucking blow your nose and wipe your eyes without getting mucous everywhere.

MICHELLE

Some people are better at harnessing the support of those closest to them to get through periods of shit. But it was easier for Michelle Yan to tell her cousins she was gay than it was to tell them she was depressed. "For the longest time, I wouldn't be able to say it. . . . It was difficult to admit to them what was happening," she tells me in the café of a north Toronto mall. And when she worked up the courage to tell them she discovered psychic pain among just about everyone else in her family. "But it was never talked about."[7]

Not in her family. Not to strangers, not to friends, not to those with whom you shared a gene pool and a home. You kept face by keeping silent. Michelle got good at keeping silent. She had realized in university that what seemed a questioning sexual uncertainty in high school was a sexual orientation, but she didn't tell her family, and it wasn't until weeks before she and her long-term girlfriend planned to move in together that Michelle told her mom she was gay.

"I very clearly remember where I was when I told her—in her bedroom. And at first she didn't really understand what I was talking about. And then when it kicked in she was like, 'That's not possible.' . . . She was devastated."

Coming out and moving out didn't make Michelle feel any less torn between the family she loved and the woman she was in love with. She agonized over her mom's response to her sexuality and struggled to explain to her girlfriend why she couldn't just tell her parents to accept her or fuck off. "She's like, 'You told her. She needs to deal with it on her own now.' And I'm like, 'I understand, but in my culture I'm very respectful toward my parents.'"

Michelle blamed herself for her mom's pain, for her girlfriend's frustration, for her own mercurial emotions that now flew out of her control, sent her bawling or yelling without warning. Even though Michelle was the primary breadwinner and caregiver while her girlfriend searched for a better job, she felt she was failing everyone she cared about most.

"We would have fights. I would threaten myself. . . . Did I want to hurt myself? I think I had serious thoughts of doing it."

She and her girlfriend broke up. Michelle moved back in with her mother. "I just completely fell apart. . . . We'd gone through so much in order for us to be together, and it had taken so long to come out to my parents, her parents. So I just thought, 'This is it, this is the be-all and end-all, for ever and ever,'" Michelle said. "And I was just like, I don't know what my life is now: my life was with her. There was no direction. . . . I couldn't see a future."

She saw a therapist, who suggested Michelle was going through depression. "I didn't want to admit it at first. I was like, what does that say about me? . . . Who would want to deal with somebody who has these types of issues? Just stacking guilt on pressure on self-blame." But ultimately, a friend going through similar angst made her see her own suffering for what it was. "He forced me to actually talk about what was going on in my head." And they'd rely on each other, each reality-checking the other's self-recrimination. "And that helped me, tremendously, in terms of being able to pull out of depression."

ON TOP OF EVERYTHING ELSE, depression has had a gender problem. When psychiatrists were delineating it as a mood disorder they reverse-engineered a reification—recruited people they thought were depressed and decided their symptoms were the symptoms of depression. But the people they thought were depressed were predominantly women. In part because they excluded people with addictions (which many men have), and in part because they just associated what they thought of as depression with women more than men. Vicious circle: because the people they included in their studies defining depression were overwhelmingly women, they then decided depression was an illness that overwhelmingly affected women. They created a set of symptoms in line with what they saw in women, and identified it using emotional language that women were socialized to use more readily.[8]

Creating a disease that pathologizes women, ignores men and adheres to cookie-cutter gender norms reverberates today: women still comprise the majority of the people diagnosed with depression and we still don't know how much of this disparity is due to the skewed way we started off defining depression or the self-reported way we diagnose it or the divergent ways mood disorders attack different people. Either women are more vulnerable to the maw of despair than men or we're doing something wrong in identifying those in its grip. Disproportionately pathologizing women bodes ill, and we've sure as hell seen it as a method of subjugation before.

But perhaps more damagingly, in the twenty-first century, this also likely means men in crisis aren't getting care. We tend not to see depression in dudes. In reporting out this book I had a hard time finding men willing to talk to me about their struggles with depression—men of colour, most of all. Gary Newman, a case worker in Toronto who spent his life working with troubled young Black men, had to pause and think when I asked if he knew of anyone who might want to talk to me: in all his years doing community work, he hadn't encountered anyone who'd been diagnosed with depression. "That's odd and speaks volumes," he said.[9]

The fact that men are more likely than women to kill themselves only muddies matters further. Society has created a damaging gendered dichotomy that exists outside humans' actual proclivity for dead-end despair.

MICHAEL

In the most marginalized and in the most successful we miss depression when it's staring us in the face.

When you hear someone say, "He had it all," the archetype you picture probably looks a lot like Lisa's older brother Michael. He was a superstar attorney with a beautiful wife, three beautiful kids, beautiful dogs in a beautiful house in Atlanta. Addicted only to his phone. "He was an athlete, he skied, he ran, he was a great son. A phenomenal brother. . . . Every role he did he was extraordinary. That's why this was such an unbelievable shock," Lisa said. "He was fearless."[10]

No one really believed he could have crippling depression. Not Michael himself or the doctors and therapists he saw. Not his wife, who couldn't reconcile this with the man she knew. Michael bounced between therapists and doctors and medications, "a whole array of different mood stabilizers," none of which seemed to work. "He got good care. He had good insurance, he had the money." He checked himself in to residential treatment programs—the Houston-based Menninger Clinic; a ranch in the Midwest; a facility near Los Angeles. "He didn't relate to the people," Lisa said. In these places, too, Michael's high-achieving success worked against him. Being surrounded by people wracked by addiction and isolation along with their depression made him feel he didn't belong, didn't need that kind of care. "I think sometimes they feel like they don't necessarily identify with these other people, because they don't have the same problem."

When Michael returned early from a stint at the Menninger Clinic "he came home feeling good, like he was helping other people there. A little bit of a manic thing, he thinks he's helping other people and he doesn't really need to be there. He thought he was fine. And I think they, even, somehow, thought it was okay for him to leave," Lisa said. "He would be charming, you know? And he had the gift of gab, and was very convincing. So I think he would fool people. . . . He was the man that always got dressed, you know? He would put on his suit and tie when he went to the office.

"Everyone perceived him as the problem-solver. You have a problem? Go to Michael. You need tickets to a football game and can't find them? Michael will know someone. . . . Sometimes the people that are the most successful, they can't—when they're used to being the winner and they're used to fixing things, and now something is broken and they can't fix it, yet they're doing everything they're supposed to—they take their meds, they show up for appointments and they're still not getting better, you know? That's frustrating."

Lisa calls it Michael's "non-lethal attempt," the time he overdosed on pills and was rushed to the psychiatric emerg. Nobody kept him, not even overnight. She wishes Michael and his nonplussed family had at least been given a brochure telling them about the risks of suicide and depression. "When my dog gets his teeth cleaned I get a better handout. He was in a high-risk category, and nobody bothered to say that. . . . That first time when he went, when he took the pills, how did they not take that opportunity? He came in with the family, why were they not given information?"

This went on for a while. Michael's degree of despondence ebbed and flowed. Then a bad cycling accident, followed by closing his law practice, made life much worse. "That was my brother's identity. . . . It was something he'd created." The final days of Michael's life were especially bad. He called his doctor, who upped his antidepressant dose, but he insisted he didn't have to go to hospital.

On the last morning of Michael's life his wife woke up to find him gone. He reappeared shortly after, said he'd been out walking. He looked at her funny—glassy-eyed, Lisa related, "like he wasn't really seeing" her. Michael's wife went back into their bedroom to get the dog's leash and he was gone by the time she returned; no sign of him as she headed out the door with the dog for a walk. The tenth-storey ledge from which he jumped was lined by a railing tall enough to require concerted effort to climb over. "It's not like it's just an edge where you don't have a second to think."

Lisa got the call from her nephew's wife. "I just stopped in my tracks. I really don't remember the rest of the conversation. . . . All I know is I just started screaming and screaming and screaming." She hadn't spoken to him that weekend. She'd been trying to give him space after he accused her of feeling sorry for him. "I said, 'No, I don't! I feel bad. . . . I don't pity you. You're a winner. You're going to be fine.' I was trying not to smother him."

Lisa knows what depression looks like: she went through it. She watched her dad go through it, hours sunk motionless into a living room chair. "I never really saw Michael like that. Because of who he was, as a person, nobody—I never—it was the biggest shock in my life. . . . You think the people who would kill themselves would be the lonely people, who don't have any money, don't have anything to live for. My brother had everything."

19

Through the Cracks

Brian David Geisheimer died on the train tracks near the bank of the Fraser River's twisting route through the Lower Mainland on its way from the Rockies to the Pacific. It would have been well after dark as he picked his way through the December night across the highway, a two-lane stretch passing houses on big lots and a low-slung motel nearby, through a thin stand of trees to reach the tracks themselves. But he'd been missing from the psych ward since late morning.

We know he died at 9:03 p.m.—a precision made possible by freight scheduling, which shows exactly what time the train reached him. "Multiple blunt force injury" is what they call it when a locomotive smashes into you at high speed.

Sebastien Pavit Abdi's time of death is less exact: there's a two-hour window during which the nineteen-year-old hanged himself, asphyxiating to death in his family home.

That same late April day, several hours earlier, Sarah Louise Charles threw herself to her death from her apartment ten storeys up.

All three died within a four-month period in 2014 and 2015. All killed themselves within hours of leaving, against medical advice, the same psychiatric ward at Abbotsford Regional Hospital near Vancouver, British Columbia, where they were supposed to have been receiving care and kept safe from their own overwhelming desire for death.

An inquest into their deaths found the hospital needed better protocols for assessing risk and for following through on those assessments, especially when the risk is high. It called on the health authority to improve its Code Yellow protocol, the code used for when a patient absconds, to quicken communication, tailor urgency to risk level, coordinate better with security guards, get police to ping the person's cell phone right away. To ensure, on discharge, that "the patient is not being rereleased into an environment that contains all of the same stressors that brought on acute care."[1] This seems at once intuitive and tricky, and it involves a therapeutically effective transition from inpatient to outpatient care that should be a matter of course but in reality rarely happens. The inquest also recommended mandatory "training and retraining" of mental health professionals in suicide risk assessment. According to a response sent to the coroner in the fall of 2018, Fraser Health has acted on several of these recommendations, including piloting standardized suicide screening, developing policies for sharing information with families and requesting funding to improve its patient release and transition process.[2]

Even if your patients don't walk out the door and kill themselves it isn't uncommon to lose them in the transition between inpatient and outpatient care. About a third of people discharged from psychiatric hospitals in Ontario see neither family doctor nor psychiatrist within a month of discharge. That could easily have been me, leaving hospital after a suicide attempt without so much as a follow-up appointment. By contrast, the vast majority of people discharged with a congestive heart failure diagnosis see their family doctor, a cardiologist or another specialist within a month, Paul Kurdyak tells me in his downtown office overlooking the Spadina streetcar line. It's no surprise, then, that one in ten people hospitalized for depression will be back in hospital for the same reason within a month. "It's a terrible patient outcome," he says, and it's like he's seeing in his mind's eye all these people lost to care. "But also, we're spending thousands of dollars on hospitalization [and] having one in four to one in three people drop off a cliff. . . . This is a ridiculous, wasteful scenario. But it's pretty common."[3]

In her work at the National Institute of Mental Health (NIMH) brain bank, Melanie Bose's postmortem detective work digging into brain donors' psychological pathologies gives her a rear-view glimpse at all the missed medical connections—records of hospital discharges with no indication of a follow-up appointment; therapeutic fits and starts with no lasting treatment. She has seen those cracks up close, in her work at a psychiatric hospital almost two decades earlier. It's not enough to schedule a follow-up appointment when someone is discharged (which not every hospital does anyway). "It depends on how motivated the person is to seek treatment, how much they like the provider, how close they are to their house, [whether] you're too depressed to have the energy." You need more of a nudge. "Just sending a brief message in the mail, you know, after a certain amount of time, they've shown that practice actually leads to lowered risk."[4]

Yes. A mailout, so that along with flyers for pizza and realtors and gym memberships is a little note saying, "Hey, how are you doing? We hope you're okay. If not, if you have questions or want to chat, give us a shout or drop by. Here's the phone number, the address, the hours. Here's how to reach us by transit."

I've gotten snail mail asking for donations to hospitals that had discharged me weeks earlier. The literal least they could do is include a little "Hey, are you thinking of killing yourself?" note.

It's easy to imagine that people who die preventable deaths were far removed from the protective embrace of society, outside the reach of any safety net—beyond help. That's a comforting lie: before people kill themselves, before they deteriorate, self-isolate, become incapacitated ciphers, they have family and friends and colleagues. Most, even when their illness begins to hijack and torment their brains, do interact with the institutions whose purpose is to get them well. Brian Ahmedani—director of Behavioral Health Services research at the Henry Ford Health System in Detroit, who was smart and kind and generous with his time—tugged threads backward to look at the histories of people who'd killed themselves and found that 83 percent of the 5,894 people in eight states he tracked over a ten-year period had contact with the health care system in the year before they killed themselves; half in their final twenty-eight days. One-fifth had a mental health–related visit in the four weeks before they killed themselves but most had no indication of a mental health problem in any health visit over that period of time. Everyone in the study had health insurance. All were "patients in well-resourced health systems." All took their own lives.[5]

What strikes Ahmedani isn't the close and frequent contact that people sucked into despair have had with the health system—"often people reach out for help right before a suicide attempt"—what strikes him is the way the system missed them. And of the myriad ways to lose people to treatable conditions, perhaps the most basic is when they're right in front of you. People are going untreated not because they aren't seeking medical care but because clinicians aren't really *seeing* the patient. And that's huge.[6]

"That, to me, is the most surprising thing," he tells me by phone. "They're reaching out—almost everyone's making some sort of visit—but either people aren't presenting symptoms right before they die, and it's just very impulsive, or we're just completely missing it. And I suspect it's a little bit of both."

This is where the Zero Suicide strategy comes in. Pioneered in the early 2000s at the Henry Ford Health System where Ahmedani is doing his groundbreaking research, it focuses on catching people at risk of suicide who are already in a health system. The version that's now being adopted around the world has seven components: to lead like you mean it; to train your workforce to spot and mitigate suicide risk; to screen, at every opportunity, for that risk, and to build those screenings into your workflow; to engage people at risk with safety plans where they outline what they'll do if shit gets real; to treat suicidality with care that's been shown to work; to transition people in a way that ensures they don't fall through the cracks between inpatient and outpatient, between one clinician and another; and to track your progress and improve upon it.[7]

Sounds obvious. It isn't.

"It really became, in my view, quite transformational for the department in how we thought about care," said Cathrine Frank, chair of Psychiatry and Behavioral Health at Henry Ford. "When we set the goal there was pushback from our staff. . . . 'How could you set a goal that is impossible?' People worried about lawsuits; they worried about not being able to deal with it. And when you really came to look at it, well, if zero isn't the goal what would the goal be? It's my relative, your friend, your teacher. It became transformational as we talked about it."[8]

Brian Ahmedani also underscores the need to screen for depression and suicide in all kinds of health encounters, because most people who kill themselves won't have gotten mental health care but will have gotten some other kind of care in the year before they die. If you don't look out for them in other health realms, he told me, they're lost.

This assumes the patient you're screening for suicide is willing to talk to you about their desire to die. Before my first attempt and in the weeks following, I certainly wouldn't have told anyone. I didn't trust clinicians. I didn't trust myself. I didn't believe my wish for oblivion was treatable, so why put myself through well-meaning interventions when honesty could very well get me locked in a hospital? I've gotten better at acknowledging and talking about my desire for death and attempts to fulfill it, but I've never been more intent on denying my suicidality than while deepest in its grip and most intent on following through.

Maybe the tired-eyed psychiatrist who assessed me that first Saturday morning in the psych emerg, who didn't know I'd been brought in against my will, who discharged me with a prescription for sleeping pills I overdosed on the next day, maybe she wasn't seeing the suicidal person in front of her. Or maybe I was dissembling too well— so intent on breaking free I convinced even myself that I was fine.

"The hardest ones to treat are the ones who've just made a decision and they aren't going to give you a clue about their plan," Jane Pearson, the head of Adult Preventive Intervention and chair of the Suicide Research Consortium at NIMH, tells me over the phone— she's among those at the forefront of tackling and somehow slowing or reversing the freaky spike in American suicides. "Fortunately, that's not the majority of people."[9]

When she says screening should be everywhere, she means it. Even when the person you're broaching it with is a child. "People are really scared when kids talk about this. And then they're like, 'Does this kid really know what they're saying?' . . . So the challenge here is trying to identify that risk and understand it more."

FAMILY PHYSICIANS ARE supposed to be your first point of contact for depression just like anything else. That's why it's called primary care.

So it's imperative GPs know how to diagnose and treat mental illness, how to assess when their patients need specialized care, and how to connect them to that care. But when it comes to severe mental illness, they may not have the knowledge and familiarity they need, says Mark Olfson, a psychiatrist at Columbia University, when I bug him with questions. "When you survey primary care doctors and you ask them which specialty they have the hardest time referring patients to, or have the hardest time identifying resources for, mental health comes to the top of the list," he says. "They're not set up to provide the level of intensity and the specialization of treatment that a lot of these more complex problems demand."[10]

Then there's the money question. Family doctors often lack the financial incentives to take the time to deal with complex, challenging, miserable patients.

Most health systems in both Canada and the US are based on a fee-for-service model, which means your family doc has an incentive to see as many patients as possible. The more patients in, or the more discrete tasks performed, the more money they make. They're also flooded with patients sporting an array of maladies, from sniffles to sepsis. It's tough to take time to probe someone's psyche, let alone attempt psychotherapy.

That's not a good enough excuse, Brian Ahmedani tells me. If someone comes in for a cold and screens positive for suicide, "what's the most important condition there? Should we really be all that worried about a cold if four days later a person's not going to be alive anymore?"

And once you do the clinical questioning and someone screens positive for depression or suicidality, what then? In many jurisdictions, you're in trouble. Your patient's in a system ill-equipped to help them, that only has resources for the well-resourced.

JAVED ALLOO'S ETHNICALLY, culturally, linguistically diverse patient population in north Toronto has worse access to mental health care now, the family doctor figures, than they've had in fifteen years. I spoke with him about how he gets his complex patients care, as a GP, and it's alarming to hear he often can't.

"It's honestly so bad now, it's scary. It's worlds worse." His frustration is palpable. "A decade or so ago, I could get someone in to see a psychiatrist in two weeks if I needed to." Now, if he has a patient who needs to see a specialist "it's pretty much: I'm going to be seeing you for the next eight months because there's nobody else who's going to be able to see you."[11] Or he's had patients referred back to him after spending a week as psychiatric inpatients—individuals "who were well beyond my capacity of care. . . . Even reading the psychiatrist's notes, I can see the challenges they're facing. And they're like, 'Okay, now I'm transferring this patient back to you."

About half his patients have coverage that pays for at least some private psychotherapy; the other half is essentially out of luck. He rarely refers patients to see psychiatrists or counsellors on an outpatient basis "because [the specialists] don't have the capacity."

When his patients' problems are beyond his scope but he can't refer them elsewhere in this fiscal year or even the next, he subs out the specialization he can't provide for the sense of stability he can. "Knowing that they have something . . . helps the safety feeling, internally."

Javed Alloo attributes his focus on patients with mental illness to his rotation in a psychiatric hospital in Kingston, Ontario, early in his career, and his work years later in an urgent-care clinic. It made him revise his idea of professional success. One of the soul-destroying things about caring for someone with a chronic condition is that you never win. Even if your patient achieves remission, depression's spectre never fully dissipates. Much of the time you're just trying to prevent irreversible decline. Maybe you can alleviate a heartbeat's worth of agony. Maybe you can help a family deal with someone who'll never get better. So your goal (to use an alliteration clinicians love) becomes "care rather than cure." Alloo remembers his grandfather having talks about death with all the grandchildren at a very young age, and how those talks helped him learn to accept early on what he can't change, and tackle all he can.

"The expectations of what you've achieved, what you're looking for as a win, changes. And as long as you can perceive the win differently, then you can say, 'This is worth my effort.'"

He figures most family physicians feel comfortable managing "relatively simpler cases of depression and suicidality." It's when people don't respond to first-, second-, even third-line treatment; when they relapse repeatedly to the point where day-to-day functioning is impaired, that he needs backup from someone with more expertise.

And that's where things often fall apart.

20

Mental Health Is for Rich People

As far as national chauvinisms go, Canada loves being The One With Universal Health Care. But if your illness is in your brain, that universality is a lie.

In theory, in Canada, psychotherapy is paid for with public dollars if you get it from a doctor—a GP or a psychiatrist or similar. I was mind-meltingly fortunate to have a psychiatrist I first saw as an inpatient and who continues to see me as an outpatient, whose invaluable sessions are covered by Ontario's public health care system. In practice, that seldom happens, and psychologists and other therapists aren't covered. People who lack private insurance or can't afford to pay out of pocket are out of luck.

In the years following the implementation of the Affordable Care Act, a higher percentage of Americans had something resembling adequate drug and psychotherapy coverage than Canadians.[1] North of the longest loosely guarded border in the world, unless you are extremely old or extremely poor or have your own plan (through your employer, for example), drugs tend not to be covered. Psychotherapy tends not to be covered, and when it is, it's near-unattainable. The only thing public dollars consistently pay for is crisis care—the costliest, least efficacious way to treat any kind of mental disorder. Post-crisis, post-discharge, you're on your own, and chances are good you'll end up needing urgent intervention again shortly.

All too often, in both Canada and the United States, if you don't have cash, mental health care isn't there.

This is often true even if you have insurance: the kind of coverage you have can determine what happens to you when you show up at the emergency room, Mark Olfson, the thoughtful Columbia University psychiatrist, told me. People on Medicaid, the insurance provided to low-income Americans, are more likely to be discharged and sent home; people with private insurance are more likely to get mental health evaluations in the emergency department and are more likely to be admitted.[2]

But this may be an indication of the resources available in the places people are accessing care rather than an indictment of doctors giving different attention to people based on their means. "The Medicaid people," Olfson tells me, "are probably going to hospitals in areas of the country where there are very few inpatient beds and there are long lines and so forth. And they're sent home, sometimes without even getting a mental health evaluation. So they're getting a lower level of care for what's ostensibly the same thing. I don't think it's the individual doctor saying, 'Well, if you have Medicaid I'm not going to provide you with a mental health evaluation.' That's not the way doctors operate. But they do operate in environments where they have varying numbers of demands on their time. They end up practising in very different ways."[3]

Inequitable insurance coverage can shaft you as an outpatient as well. In the United States, psychiatrists are significantly less likely than other medical specialists to accept any kind of insurance—private or public. The greater your financial need the less likely it is that the psychiatrist nearest you will take whatever coverage you have. Just over half of American psychiatrists accept private insurance; but just 43 percent accept Medicaid—far lower than for non-psychiatric clinicians. And psychiatrists are less likely to accept insurance than they were a decade ago.[4] That means you either have to pay cash or go elsewhere.

"That's a really huge problem," Maria Oquendo, past president of the American Psychiatric Association and chair of psychiatry at the

University of Pennsylvania's Perelman School of Medicine, tells me when I call her, seeking clarity. In many cases, she adds, it's because insurers undervalue behavioural health care, reimbursing psychiatrists so little it isn't worth their time. "An insurer here in Philadelphia pays $44 for a ten-minute consultation. You can't get a plumber to show up for that, you know what I mean? So it puts doctors in a very difficult bind."[5]

Mental health care is what economists call "price-sensitive"— cost changes, even small ones, can determine whether you get it or not. "It's an interesting dynamic," Tim Bruckner, who is an epidemiologist and public health professor, tells me in his office at the University of California, Irvine, where I'd sought him out because of his work on how public health measures change who gets or needs what kind of care. "If you break your arm it doesn't really matter what the cost of the X-ray is: you're basically going [to hospital to get one]. If the price of antidepressants drops by 10 percent, or psychiatric care drops, you seek more care."[6] That price includes travel, wait times and myriad indignities and inconveniences that can deter people from getting care for their minds that they otherwise might.

Variable quality of mental health care can be an issue in public systems, too. Barely half of the 108,000 British Columbians in Professor Joseph Puyat's study at the University of British Columbia, all of whom had a depression diagnosis for which they were receiving public health care, received "minimally adequate" treatment. Even if you get your foot in the door, poorer people are more likely to get "poor or under-treatment by any published standard."[7]

So that's bad.

On top of everything else, you need to learn to make a fuss. If you don't, no matter how your care's paid for—private insurance, public insurance, out of pocket—you may get passed over or rushed through when you need something more. If my parents hadn't pushed for a second opinion that, frankly, I didn't want, I'd have been discharged post-suicide attempt with negligible follow-up. Being pushy takes determination and time and a degree of confidence in the system and your place in it. People who are marginalized in other aspects of their lives—by race, by income, by language, by immigration status—are less likely to have that confidence.

And the people least able to haggle effectively are those with the most severe mental illness—either because they lack the wherewithal to do so or they don't think anything will make them better or they simply don't believe they deserve care. Or because their haggling isn't effective—it's easy to dismiss a crazy person's kvetching no matter how justified. I've spoken to so many people who felt they weren't heard, weren't listened to when making concerns known. I've been in that position, talking to a nurse's receding back. It's a great way to deny meaningful care in the short term and ensure it won't be sought in the long term.

So you give up. You get sicker. You don't know whom to call, where to turn to advocate for yourself when you can't get an appointment with someone who'll treat you. Maybe things get bad enough you end up in a psychiatric ER and maybe you get some helpful treatment there but chances are you get no follow-up afterward.

More psychiatrists would help but that wouldn't be enough: a study that Paul Kurdyak authored from Toronto in 2014 found that psychiatrists in urban areas—where they're most highly concentrated—tend to keep seeing the same few patients rather than taking in new ones. Psychiatrists in Toronto saw 57 percent fewer new outpatients than psychiatrists in areas with a far smaller supply of shrinks per capita.[8] "A small number of people have access to that kind of intensive service [that psychiatrists in urban areas offer] and many more are making do with either nothing or primary care," he tells me.[9]

I am an abashed beneficiary of this service inequity: living in Toronto, I see my psychiatrist as an outpatient on a weekly basis. This luxury no doubt steals time that could otherwise go to sick people waiting weeks or months to see someone. But I *like* seeing my psychiatrist on a regular basis. If the goal is my continuing to function and work and not die, I *need* to—these appointments are the only thing consistently giving me hope.

Should there be visit frequency limits? Different pay scales? Psychiatrists designated as intake physicians for new patients? Would it help if psychiatrists were more closely associated with hospitals? Jury's still out on that. Ontario tried to incentivize psychiatrists to see more urgent patients by offering a bonus to those who'll see patients who've recently been discharged from hospital or tried to kill themselves. But results were mixed. And according to Kurdyak: "Collectively, we have a responsibility to meet a need."

He'd like to see clustered mental health care teams combining practitioners from different disciplines, with a triage-like structure in place to determine who goes where to get what care, and where they go next.

South of the border, Michael Schoenbaum, as a senior advisor on the economics of mental care at the National Institute of Mental Health (NIMH), has been pushing Collaborative Care. I called him at the suggestion of NIMH's Jane Pearson. "Everyone says they collaborate; that's not what this means."[10]

Schoenbaum comes at mental health care as an economist, trying to get his head around why we keep failing at getting basic, necessary interventions to people who need them.

"We have these existing treatments that are a lot better than nothing, even if they are not everything we would want them to be. But quite a high fraction of people with depression don't receive anything."

Right now, your family doctor diagnoses you with depression, sends you home with an antidepressant prescription. Maybe you're instructed to come back if things get worse. How much worse is worse? What if worse means losing the will to bug people to help you halt and reverse that spiral? Initiating an intervention and then leaving the person being intervened upon to their own devices is bad in any field of health care, Schoenbaum says, but it's especially bad in a condition characterized by floundering in isolation and a reluctance or inability to seek help. "This traditional medical model of, you know, tell the patient what to do and then leave it to the patient to come back and self-identify if they're having a problem and ask for something different, just works really badly." In his model, someone follows up. A health care coordinator—someone who doesn't need to be an MD or even a health specialist—calls you a few weeks after your initial appointment to see how you're doing—confirming you filled the prescription or followed up on whatever else was prescribed, confirming you're taking it as directed, that it's working, that the side effects are tolerable. "If the patient isn't getting better, again, you reach out to the patient, say, 'Look, we started you on this thing. We need to do better: this isn't working for you. Let's bring you back in.'"

And perhaps more important than that patient-clinician liaison is a clinician-clinician link. Doctors talking to each other. That's the idea behind Collaborative Care.

In principle, right now, when a general practitioner feels they're in over their head in treating a particular patient's malady, they'll refer that patient to a specialist for a consult. Sometimes, a clinician will hesitate to do that because they don't know when they're in over their head or, far more likely, because they know the patient will spend months waiting for that consult. Many non-specialists are hesitant to even ask if you want to die if they don't know where they'll send you if the answer is affirmative. The idea behind Collaborative Care is that if you're a GP you can call up your psychiatrist colleague—maybe even walk down the hall and chat in person—and ask about your patient's case, whether you should switch meds or try something else, whether what you thought was unipolar depression could be bipolar. It could mean problems are caught early; it would save money and improve outcomes. Models of this exist in little bits throughout the continent: family health teams, collaborative care units, whatever you want to call them. In Ontario you can bill for calling another doctor for advice and for providing that guidance. Governments like to tout such models as indications of innovative health spending but they remain the exception, not the rule.

Right now, phone-a-colleague is not on the list of many health payers' billable items. As Michael Schoenbaum said, "Most insurers don't and wouldn't cover this specialty consultation between the primary care team and the psychiatrist."

It's a potential starting point, though—a health system with crucial connective tissue between doctor and patient, doctor and doctor. We need more, and more accessible, psychiatrists, both to provide expertise and to provide care for those people whose problems are more complex.

And if you don't want mental wellness to remain the purview of the privileged, if you don't want poverty to doom people to debilitating anguish, you need to cover pharmacotherapy and psychotherapy like you mean it. Universally. For everyone.[11]

21

Trying to Heal the Littlest Minds

Societies have a thing about children. They are precious bringers of the future, and the seat of all our anxieties. Are parents doing too much, or too little? Are teachers being too demanding, or not demanding enough? We fret over the ways they spend or don't spend their free time, and what they do or don't do with the latest technology available to them, be it video games or computers or cell phones or smartphones. Somehow, something is ruining a generation.

So it is with mental illness, where the spectre of crazy-sick kids looms large. Every year, more than three thousand North American children, teens and adolescents kill themselves. Tens of thousands more try. The US Centers for Disease Control's annual survey of high-school students found that 8.6 percent of teens said they had tried to kill themselves. Girls were more than twice as likely as boys (11.6 percent compared to 5.5 percent).[1]

And the death toll, for youth, is rising. Suicide rates among twenty- to twenty-four-year-olds increased 35 percent; twenty-five- to twenty-nine-year-olds, 34 percent. The rate for fifteen- to nineteen-year-olds increased 75 percent. The suicide rate for ten- to fourteen-year-olds more than doubled between 2007 and 2017. America's overall suicide rate increased about 26 percent between 2007 and 2017. A big jump, to be sure. But not the spike we're seeing with youth.[2]

The rise in youth suicide is shocking the world's suicide researchers and those caring for the suicidal.

"We are flabbergasted, to be quite honest," Arielle Sheftall, a research scientist at Nationwide Children's Hospital in Columbus, Ohio, admits over the phone. "When you look at the percentages in ten- to fourteen-year-olds, it has so significantly increased to the point where you go, 'Whoah, this is bad.' And in females, specifically, it's skyrocketed."[3]

Especially disturbing is her finding among the littlest attempters of suicide. The idea of a twelve-year-old taking their life churns your gut, turns it cold. So the very idea of someone as young as five or six killing themselves defies my conceptualization—even if (the good news) suicide rates among the youngest children are vanishingly small—measured in per-million, as opposed to per–hundred thousand for other age groups. But "it breaks my heart every time I talk about it. We like to think kids at that age are prospering: they're just starting school, they're becoming their own individuals."

But it happens. Kids kill themselves.

Her research found rates rising dramatically among Black kids even as they fell among white ones.

We don't know why but we can hypothesize, she says. It could be because Black children are more likely to be exposed to the kind of violence or trauma that can put them at increased risk of self-inflicted death. It could be caregivers' reluctance to seek help from institutions that have historically betrayed their trust. But this is a field of research we don't know enough about because the necessary resources have not been put in place to explore it.

EVERYONE HAS A THEORY about what's behind the rise in child and youth suicide broadly.

Madelyn Gould, an epidemiologist in psychiatry at Columbia University, tells me she worries about shifting norms—that kids see suicide as an option now when they didn't before. Decades ago, "You might be depressed, you might have serious psychiatric problems, but people wouldn't kill themselves. It happened, but it was still rare."[4]

It's easy to blame the media. It's easy to blame social media. It's easy to blame shows like *13 Reasons Why*, a Netflix series chronicling a high schooler's suicide (which I've never seen nor want to see) in which, as Gould says, "help-seeking wasn't accessible but dying by suicide was very accessible."

Norms matter. Her research shows that youth who think their peers have considered or attempted suicide are more likely to consider or attempt themselves.

Options matter. She has a problem with coverage that doesn't emphasize—to kids and caregivers—that there's help (whether help is actually available, as we've seen, obviously depends).

But the truth is, no one knows for sure what's driving this increase across the board that's especially pronounced among the youngest suicide victims, Arielle Sheftall points out.

"People will say a number of things—'It's social media, it's this, it's that' and people want to grab on to these things and believe that they're the culprits, but we don't know. We don't know. And I don't want to say, 'Yup, it's all Facebook,' because we don't know that's the case."

One thing she wants to drive home, that she repeats a couple of times during our conversation, is the need to pay attention to kids' disclosures of suicidal thoughts—no matter how jokey or flippant they seem. "Statements like, 'Oh, I just want to die' may come off as 'funny,' quote-unquote, but the kid might really mean that. And if we don't address that, how can we get them the help they need?"

People are afraid to have those conversations with anyone, let alone a little kid. Shit, I'd be terrified of mentioning it. Arielle Sheftall says I shouldn't be. Maybe I'd be more likely to do so, though, if I knew what to do if the answer was affirmative. Jane Pearson, the suicide-prevention expert with NIMH, has said primary care clinicians are more likely to ask if you're suicidal if they know where to send you if you say yes, and I don't doubt it's the same, if not more so, for the layperson.[5]

IT'S BAD FOR YOUTH, and it's especially bad for some kids of colour, but suicidality seems to be worse for LGBTQ youth. Three in ten queer high-school students attested to having tried to kill themselves in the past year—more than quadruple the rate of straight students. One in ten made a suicide attempt so serious it needed medical attention.[6] The Centers for Disease Control's study makes no mention of trans youth, which is telling. We know trans young people are also at elevated risk of trying to kill themselves, and evidence suggests similar factors around rejection and discrimination are at play.[7]

It's harder to know for sure whether gender and sexual minorities are more likely to die by suicide; that kind of data tends not to be collected at the medical examiner level, and studies involving individual-level psychological autopsies have been inconclusive. But the relationship between sexual orientation, gender identity and non-fatal suicidal behaviour is much clearer, and has been found in North America, Europe, Australasia and elsewhere.[8]

I called Ann Haas, a veteran suicidologist with the kind of deep voice you'd want narrating your documentary, to figure out how it's possible that we know so little about the risk of suicide to a group of people we know to be at heightened risk of trying to kill themselves.

She and her colleagues at the American Foundation for Suicide Prevention designed a way to ascertain and record a person's gender and sexual orientation in death reports, but the catch is you need to do it in every single death or your records are of little use. And uptake has been scant.

America remains squeamish about sex and gender to a damaging degree, she said.

Haas, who is lesbian, found herself drawn to the study of LGBTQ suicidality—especially among young people—because of what she saw in her own community.

"I just saw so many people struggling and it seemed like a different pattern—it just never quite seemed like it fit with what we knew about other groups. And the more I work with these populations the more convinced I am that there are some very unique factors that are driving suicidal behaviour. And at the same time, we know so little."[9]

Among those factors is discrimination, and the way it erases your stability and your selfhood. LGBTQ people living in US states without protections against discrimination reported higher prevalences of mood, anxiety and substance disorders compared with straight people in those states or gay people in other states that boasted better protections.[10] A similar trend was found in the wake of state bans on same-sex marriage following the 1996 Defense of Marriage Act—even in states that didn't enact bans themselves but where homophobic rhetoric made itself felt.[11]

One study of lesbian, gay and bisexual-identifying individuals in New York City found that while white participants had higher rates of mood disorders, Black and Latino individuals had higher rates of suicide attempts. This could be because suicide attempts among queer people of colour are more related to external stressors than internal disorders;[12] or it could be because we're bad at recognizing mood disorders in people who aren't white.

WE'RE SCARED OF making kids crazy and we're scared of giving kids crazy pills, and in 2004 when the US Food and Drug Administration mandated warning labels on antidepressants cautioning clinicians that they could make kids want to kill themselves, it reverberated. The fine print of the precipitating analysis,[13] which found an almost doubled prevalence of suicidality among kids on antidepressants versus placebo, is worth noting: the trials included in the analysis weren't designed to measure suicide risk; and they focused on ideation, not attempted or completed suicides.

The black box warning and the scary headlines it brought had a significant impact.[14] In the years immediately following, antidepressant prescribing for kids and adolescents dropped sharply after having risen for several years, even as the number of self-poisonings with psychotropic drugs rose and other kinds of depression treatment stayed stagnant.[15]

It would be too simplistic to attribute the spike in youth suicides to black box warnings fifteen years ago. But if they played even a small role in making doctors reluctant to treat depression in youth, that's damaging.[16]

There are some risk factors we know about, however.

Childhood trauma is one. A family history of mental illness is another. And there are ways depression manifests itself in children that make the adults in their lives more likely to miss it.

More so than adults, young people are responsive to their environments. It means the things happening to them and around them can help trigger a descent into mental illness. And it means mental illness may not manifest the way you think it does, which means it goes unnoticed or is confused with something else, Betsy Kennard, a researcher and director of Outpatient Psychological Services at UT Southwestern, informs me over the phone.

"You could have a depressed kid and put him in the computer lab and he enjoys the computer game so he might not look, to the teacher, as depressed because he's smiling and interacting. Or you have a kid who is maybe irritable and oppositional and your tendency is not to see that kid as depressed: you see them as maybe being willful and uncooperative and maybe spoiled."[17]

"Whereas depressed adults tend to have a flat affect—they will be sad in every different environment—children can show, you know, positive affect because they're doing something they like and then they go back to their routine and they may look depressed."

And many adults often have a hard time coming to grips with the possibility that their child is depressed—especially when this little person they provide for has an objectively easier childhood than they did themselves.

"Even though there's been a lot of years of work on childhood depression, it's still hard for people to really grasp that a child can be depressed. . . . It's hard to see in your child. It's hard to know what to do."

THERE ARE PEOPLE about whom the hackneyed phrase "you're stronger than you know" feels true. Maybe Marcella, raising daughters on her own on a Navajo reservation in Utah, knows it now. I hope the kickboxing helped.

MARCELLA AND BREANNA

By the time Marcella entered her daughter's room, sixteen-year-old Breanna was mottled grey-blue.[18]

It wasn't unusual for Breanna to stomp into her room in a sudden jarring rage and lock the door. It was weird, though, that there was no response when Breanna's younger sister banged on the door and yelled, when their Australian shepherd, Jake, whined outside the bedroom, agitated and disconsolate.

"He kept scratching at her door, he kept trying to crawl underneath the door and he's just whimpering and running up and down the hall and then finally he just lay down and didn't move."

It was probably around noon when they heard the big thud.

"And that's when we go back—and we always go back; me and the girls keep going back to the minute we heard that thud. 'We should have done this; we should have done that; why didn't we do this,' you know. And we go back to those woulda-coulda-shouldas."

Marcella goes back to the moment she finally got fed up and barged into Breanna's room, hours after the teen had shut herself inside. Breanna's shift at McDonald's started at three o'clock and it was unheard of for her, obsessively conscientious, to be late for work. "I actually was so mad. I was like, 'What is wrong with you, kid?' I ended up unscrewing the doorknob because for some reason I didn't want to break the door down because I didn't want to spend $70 on a new door. And that was so stupid for me to even think about that. I should have broken that door down. Seventy dollars would have been nothing. And I go back to that.

"I opened the door and that's when I saw her. She was probably less than an inch off the floor; just a little bit more and she would have, she would have made it. . . . 'You could have just wiggled just a little bit and you would have hit the floor.'"

Breanna had hanged herself from her closet by a belt her mother'd never seen before. "I was wondering, like, 'Where did this belt come from?' . . .

"The first emotion I felt when I found her was anger. At her. I mean, because my mind hadn't coped with the fact that she's gone." She took out her rage on the contents of her daughter's room— everything in the closet, band posters on the wall. "What was the point of you putting up a poster? What was that whole point if you were going to do this?"

FIVE YEARS AFTER her eldest child killed herself Marcella's pain has begun to ebb but the image still materializes, unbidden. "Cutting her down was probably the hardest thing. It comes back and comes back."

Everything Marcella didn't see now throbs, obvious—childhood trauma, cataclysms of rage, punishing self-recrimination when Breanna couldn't meet her own high standards. Breanna had been sexually assaulted when she was five years old. She started cutting herself at ten. "She would cover up with bracelets and I never saw them."

It was easy for warning signs to fly under the radar. In Marcella's family, dysfunction was the norm.

"It was a lot of domestic violence. And I think for Native Americans it's really common to see that kind of a dysfunctional family. Not only that, but noticing the alcohol that's also involved. To us, it was normal. I mean, when we were growing up. And then it's kind of like it's passed on from generation to generation."

Marcella didn't even think of it as a suicide attempt when as an adolescent she leapt from a moving car, or when, later, she overdosed on pills. "It didn't seem to me like it was that bad, in a way." And teenage Marcella "acted out." "I would get in trouble a lot with the police, and [had] a juvenile record. . . . I would always be going to court for dealing or looting or vandalism or something that, just, I can't imagine my kids doing right now."

Breanna's birth when Marcella was fifteen years old saved her, she said. "That's when reality and responsibility kicked in."

A mother of two before she turned twenty, Marcella worked full-time to cover a $300-a-month apartment. She can't imagine her own teenage daughters doing the same. "My little one, she's sixteen right now and I can't even fathom seeing her raising a little child at her age."

Marcella's partner abused her for years—"not just emotional: physical, mental, everything. . . . It got pretty severe." He never hit his children but they saw everything. Breanna, who'd always been close to her dad, felt especially conflicted. Finally, "I said, 'No. I can't do this anymore.'" But when he walked out he took most of their income with him. "He was the primary breadwinner. So there's the mortgage, there's the car payments, everything. We ended up losing everything. . . . I ended up having to get two full-time jobs, and that's when I gave [Breanna] the primary responsibility of taking care of her sisters, because I would go to work at six in the morning, get off at three thirty and go to my next job at three forty-five and get off at twelve midnight. So I never really saw my kids."

When they moved three, four times in their Utah reservation within a couple of years, Breanna was there beside her mother at two in the morning, moving their furniture while her little sisters slept. "It was a huge burden on her growing up, because I depended on her. It was like, 'Okay, Breanna, did you cook for your sisters? Breanna, did you pick up your sisters? Breanna, did you . . . ?' It was constant.

At some point she probably felt like she didn't have her own life. . . . I might have given her a bit too much responsibility for her age."

Through high school Breanna "was such a good kid"—good grades, no drugs, no booze. Long-term boyfriend. She relished the discipline of Junior Reserve Officers' Training Corps, a pre-military program for youth. "She had a path . . . she knew exactly where she wanted to go. She wanted to go to the art institute. She was going to travel the world."

It's easy, now, for her mom to see that driving perfectionism as something more ominous. "She wouldn't give herself any little bit of room to make mistakes. . . . She always had to be perfect. . . . She had so much that she wanted to do. And she piled all of that on herself."

And then there was the anger—roiling, violent outbursts out of nowhere. She'd run at her sisters with a knife at the least provocation. "I would question her, like, 'Are you okay? Are you depressed?'. . . She would brush it off." The outbursts intensified in the last months and weeks of her life. A group of girls beat her up to the point her mom transferred her to another school. She had a wrenching argument with one of her best friends.

The summer morning of her death featured an escalating fight over the most seemingly minor things: Marcella, hungover from the night before, was slower to get up to register Breanna for school that fall. Breanna was anxious and angry at the prospect of spending her own hard-earned money for new tires on her car. "I think she just made herself even more upset just thinking about all of that. So we had an argument and she ended up slamming the door in my face" so hard that picture frames toppled off the wall.

Breanna's final text was to her boyfriend at around 11:50 a.m. "I'm doing it now."

He didn't freak out: she'd said that before. Marcella says he told her later: "'I didn't take her seriously because she didn't do it the last couple of times.' I never knew."

In the immediate aftermath of Breanna's suicide, "I don't remember even being. I don't even remember what time or the hours or the days were. . . . I noticed that time would pass because the flowers were beginning to die."

For the first time she found herself seeking psychological help for herself and her family. She barely knew where to start. Her younger girls went to a child-centred counselling group but found it alienating to be around kids talking about uncles' or grandparents' accidental or natural deaths when their hurt felt so much worse.

"We didn't know how to cope. We didn't know how to get back to normal. . . . It's a pain that is so indescribable. It's like your body is trying to find a way to fix it and fix it and there's no way that it's ever going to be fixed."

For a year Marcella was in the depths of depression. "I kind of had no motivation to work anymore. I couldn't." She used her employer's family medical leave "because I felt I was not worthy to even work. I felt that I was not worthy of anything."

Counselling for herself and her girls is more obtainable now than it was several years ago, she says. "Back then it was really hard to get it on your insurance. You had to go through several evaluations and you also had to get a referral in order for you to see a psychiatrist or any kind of mental health [practitioner]. . . . We had to go through hoops and ladders in order for us to get to see anyone."

Kickboxing helped, from an anger-expunging perspective. So did the reminder she still had two living girls to care for. Fear her daughters will emulate their older sister keeps Marcella on alert, changed her parenting. Puts work second, now, always. "After the suicide I began to start coddling my children—my kids that are alive now. . . . It feels almost like you're walking on eggshells. Like, 'Okay, I don't want to make this mistake again. What am I going to do different so I don't make this mistake again?' And it's awful, because it's a guilty feeling."

"It's easy to say" that it's not her fault, Marcella tells me, a uselessly empathic reporter. "I think that's what we all struggle with."

Her daughter's death granted her involuntary entry to a world of suicide she hadn't known existed. "I wasn't introduced to suicide when I was younger. . . . I had two family members, before my daughter passed away, that had committed suicide. And nobody in my family ever shared that with me. It was like a hidden secret." An aunt overdosed on pills. A cousin drowned himself and his mom couldn't countenance it. Even after her other son was found hanging, strangled, years later, she still would not acknowledge what had killed them.

"She won't talk about it. . . . I can't ask her, 'How did it feel?' She lost her kids—both her kids—to the same thing. . . . And she won't talk about it. She won't acknowledge it at all."

Now Marcella derives purpose from smashing that walled unwillingness to confront suicide.

"My role now is I need to make sure that people are aware of this and people understand what this can do to a family if it's not talked about."

Now she has friends come to her for advice. She's often the only person they'll tell. "One of them had a son that was beginning to cut himself and he started to leave notes for his dad saying he's going to do this. And he approached me, he asked me, 'What should I do? What should I listen to?'

"It is really huge on the reservation. Nobody wants to talk about it. Nobody wants to say, 'Oh yeah, they took their own life.' And nobody sees that there's a need to heal that pain. They just bear it and the pain is passed on and they just bear it and bear it and bear it and basically it ends up eating them up. . . . I was guilty of that, too. Because the first two years [after] her passing away I didn't acknowledge her suicide. I didn't even tell people that she killed herself. I just said it was an accident or I wouldn't really go into it. It's something that needs to be talked about. Because if we don't say anything, nobody is going to say anything, and nobody's going to understand anything. And, to me, I felt I had a personal responsibility to make sure that nobody else goes through this."

• • •

AGAIN AND AGAIN and again, I find, the people who feel most keenly depression's and suicide's toll are those who've been there. It hits home for Arielle Sheftall, who now researches child suicide: she was fourteen years old when her mom died and her world just about fell apart. "It was a very, very tough time. And thoughts of suicide, absolutely. I would have thoughts of suicide." But she was lucky, she says: she told an older cousin who got her the help she needed.

The knowledge that not everyone has that luck helps drive her.

"I've kind of lived that experience and I just want to, from my own experience, help others and say, 'There is a light at the end of the tunnel. And there is a lot that's unknown, but there are things we do know that do work. And if that doesn't work, maybe we try this. . . . So, I think," she says to me, "that's why suicide really is one of the topics that I'm very passionate about.

"It's something that hits home, but it's preventable."

22

"More Children Do Not Have to Die"

Human beings have a finite capacity for outrage and at some point Canadians ran out of outrage at twelve-year-olds across the country killing themselves for lack of care. It was the litany, I think—one child suicide after another, sometimes in suicide pacts, in Indigenous communities few could find on a map, in situations that boggle belief and numb the mind. States of emergency became constants but the urgency never seemed to last long enough to produce lasting change; inaction left crises unaddressed and robbed those crises of their power. And it was the degree of systemic deprivation behind the awfulness—not just lack of mental health care but also lack of housing and clean water and opportunities for hope, and the legacy of residential schools and centuries of concerted genocidal attempts to stamp out entire peoples and their cultures.

JOLYNN

Kerri Cutfeet met his daughter for the first time when she was twelve years old in the cafeteria of Thunder Bay hospital's pediatric psych ward. Jolynn Winter had been there two weeks after running away from her foster home—the latest of many foster homes in small communities all over Northern Ontario. Just weeks earlier, in the wake of a close friend's suicide, she'd tried to hang herself with a T-shirt from a bathroom stall coat hook. While she was held as an inpatient—"they just locked her up in there"—in a city where she knew no one, her case worker at Tikinagan Child and Family Services was calling around, trying to find her somewhere to live.[1]

Kerri was living with his partner and two young kids on the Wapekeka First Nation reserve in Northern Ontario, a fly-in community hundreds of kilometres from the nearest mid-sized city. He'd discovered Jolynn was his daughter just four years earlier, he told me, but had kept his distance: she was enmeshed in the foster system and he wasn't sure she'd appreciate this stranger inserting himself into her life. Now, though, was different. Now the eldest child he'd never met needed a home.

"My partner, she said, 'Kerri, you should do something, already.' . . . Hearing that, from her, that was awesome."

It took all of a week to sort everything out. He met with Jolynn's caseworker to hammer out a plan for when she was released—the structure she would need, what he would provide, the options she would have if she needed additional care.

And then Kerri was in the Thunder Bay Regional Health Centre psych-ward cafeteria. Terrified.

"I was so nervous and so scared but so excited. I was afraid she was pissed off at me—disappointed in me, you know? For not being there all her life. She didn't even really look at me right away. And she kind of gave me this nervous smile and I got up and hugged her and I texted my partner right away, as soon as I seen her, just saying, 'Oh, she's beautiful.'"

They went from the hospital to the mall, where Kerri bought Jolynn a winter jacket and a rose-gold-coloured heart-shaped necklace, then flew home, where they had a room of her own all ready for her.

His younger children, nine and ten, were ecstatic at the prospect of a brand-new older sister. "What I felt so bad about was that one question: 'Where was she all our lives?' . . . They were just so happy to have her."

He remembers, right away, trying to talk to Jolynn—about herself, and what she'd been through; about her mom, and why she'd ultimately had to give Jolynn up to family services; about why he hadn't gotten in touch earlier. "Anything to make her feel better."

And she was happy, he said.

It wasn't until afterward that he learned she'd stopped calling her doctor and her caseworker after she moved in.

Kerri's voice glows when he talks about the way Jolynn became comfortable with him, made demands of him a daughter would of her dad. "She'd text us and say something along the lines of, 'One of you come and get me while one of you starts cooking! I'm hungry!'" The thing she requested most was cupcakes. "And then, as she got more comfortable with me, she'd say, 'Get me cupcakes!' That felt good, you know? She didn't ask, she demanded."

Christmas was a joy. A house full of children and Xboxes and children squabbling good-naturedly over Xboxes. By winter break Jolynn had already made friends and Kerri figured it was cool for her to stay out a bit later—there was no school to worry about waking up for. And he knew readjusting after the holidays to the schedule they'd agreed to follow would be a challenge. He tried to nudge Jolynn gently toward self-discipline. "My very last message to her on Facebook . . . I told her, 'It's about time that you start coming in earlier, sleeping earlier, because you've got to go to school. We both signed a paper saying we would follow that safety plan.' That was part of it, going to school."

There was another death, right when school was starting up again: Jolynn's cousin in Lac Seul, several hundred kilometres away, was found frozen to death outside one morning. Jolynn wouldn't talk about it, Kerri said.

"She must have taken it pretty hard. She said she was sad about it but I didn't see her expressing it, you know?"

His daughter didn't express sadness much at all, for that matter. The only time he'd seen her cry was at a silly video her friend posted on Facebook. She laughed and laughed but suddenly was sobbing.

"And I asked her, 'What are you laughing about?' And she said, 'I'm not laughing, I'm crying.'"

But she seemed happy, he said. He did everything he could so she'd be happy.

They'd developed a morning routine: he'd get up and sit on the couch and watch her bedroom door, which opened out to the living room.

"She'd poke her head out, look around and then scurry to the washroom. And every morning I'd wait for that to happen."

"I didn't want to go bug her—she was a young lady and I didn't want to invade her space too much. But I'd make sure I heard something, at least. Like, if I didn't hear anything from the room for a while I'd go knock or something and say, 'Hey, what's up?'"

That Sunday, Kerri decided to sleep in. Didn't rush to the couch to check for that head poking out, for the scurrying out to the washroom. It wasn't until close to two o'clock that his partner's shriek yanked him awake.

He raced through the living room to Jolynn's bedroom door and saw his partner on the floor, Jolynn in her arms. A string—a shoelace, he thinks, or the pullstring of a hoodie—tight around her neck. She'd hanged herself, sitting, from the doorknob. Her body's weight had pulled the door ajar, which is when Kerri's partner saw her. And screamed.

"I could still feel some life in her, but just barely. She was all pale, there was no colour to her skin, and she was all blue and purple around the mouth and lips."

He cut the string off, started CPR, did whatever he could think of to try and breathe life back into his blueing daughter.

And, hysterical, called the clinic—a nursing station that would send paramedics round in an emergency. The agonizing slowness of their response hasn't lessened in his mind. It took an eternity for a driver to come, an eternity for him to come in, to try to resuscitate his little girl. He covered his two younger children's eyes to try to spare them the image of their sister's strangulation, the way the sight of an uncle's suicide had burned itself into his eight-year-old brain decades earlier. "I just didn't want my kids to have that image."

They finally put Jolynn in the back of the truck and brought her to the clinic, to try to save her there. For hours they tried, before pronouncing her dead.

Later he learned she was bullied online—messages telling her, "Kill yourself." And that she was part of a suicide pact with a number of other young girls from the community—a pact community leaders had gone to the federal government to try to stop. Months later, her brother, ten years old, was a target: "This person made a video about my son, poking fun at him, telling him to kill himself, too. . . . It might even be the same person. I don't even know."

There's no good way to ask a dad what could have kept his little girl alive. Would it have helped her to have supports in the community—a therapist, a doctor?

"I'm not sure about that. There were people to talk to."

TWO DAYS AFTER twelve-year-old Jolynn Winter hanged herself from her bedroom doorknob on a Sunday in January 2017, her friend Chantell Fox, also twelve, took her own life. Both were members of the four-hundred-person Wapekeka First Nation. All suicides are preventable tragedies but theirs feel particularly so because they were predicted. Jolynn and Chantell were both part of the suicide pact community leaders had discovered six months earlier, prompting a plea for funds—$376,706 for salaries, benefits, training and rent for a four-person suicide prevention team. "There have been many suicide attempts by youth in the past year and it is believed that there is a suicide pact with a group of young females," reads the request, submitted to the Canadian federal government, which is responsible for health care on reserves, in July 2016.[2]

The proposal met with radio silence save for rote acknowledgement from Health Canada.

Days after Jolynn's and Chantell's suicides, Nishnawbe Aski Nation grand chief Alvin Fiddler called out Canada's prime minister Justin Trudeau for his inaction in a letter all the more damning for its lack of bombast.

> *I write not to embarrass you, not simply to make a political point, but to plead for the sake of our youth and, as a matter of life and death, that you immediately act on these solutions. . . .*
>
> *Canada has run out of excuses for these tragedies.*[3]

Trudeau met with Grand Chief Fiddler and other Indigenous leaders; was reportedly "receptive" to their ideas but short on promises.

And then in June, twelve-year-old Jenera Roundsky killed herself shortly after returning home to Wapekeka after spending months in a residential treatment facility hundreds of kilometres away. The community had opposed her discharge, said Wapekeka council member Joshua Frogg, who was Chantell's uncle and who, in the wake of the preteen suicides, became something of a community spokesperson.[4]

These girls were Michael Kirlew's patients.

In an affidavit before Canada's Human Rights Tribunal that year, the family doctor laid responsibility for the children's suicides on government failure to provide basic health care—preventive or urgent—to these kids and their communities.

"In my daily medical practice, I can draw a direct correlation between the lack of access to *early* medical interventions leading to compounded mental health problems and youth suicide. . . . This recent suicide crisis in Wapekeka is not the first suicide crisis that has occurred and I fear that it will not be the last suicide crisis if the status quo remains. Wapekeka has routinely identified what they need to address the high rate of youth suicide. These tragedies are preventable and more *children* do not need to die."[5]

This is one small remote community.

Similar scenes play out in Indigenous homes across the continent.

Stateside, Native American children aged ten to seventeen are killing themselves at a rate 62 percent higher than white people of the same age. The disparity is worse for adolescent girls, who are killing themselves at almost three times the rate of their white counterparts and whose suicide rate increased almost 90 percent between 1999 and 2015. The suicide rate for eighteen- to twenty-four-year-old girls more than doubled in that time and has been, consistently, more than double the average. (Among young Indigenous boys the suicide rate, while still higher than average, has dropped or stayed steady.)[6] And these are probably significant underestimations, because deaths of Indigenous Americans tend to go under-reported.[7]

It's easy to lose hope, to feel the systemic injustices plaguing North America's Indigenous communities are too deep-rooted to tackle. But the people making the most difference in that epidemic of despair are Indigenous communities themselves, picking up the slack left by government bodies that are actually responsible for providing services. Or look at the We Matter campaign—because that needs saying!—a Canadian initiative started by Indigenous youth meant to instill a sense of hope where it's lacking.[8] Countless organizations and initiatives seek to fill in the fatal cracks too many people fall through.

GORDON POSCHWATTA GOT a suicide call while we were talking on the phone.

Luckily he was already in his car on his way to Burns Lake, partway through that day's two-hundred-odd-kilometre odyssey from one remote British Columbia community to another. Unseasonably muddy November roads made a long journey longer. "I'm gonna blame today on global warming," he says from the side of the road, where he's pulled over to chat in a pocket of forest with decent mobile reception. I can hear the quiet clicking of his hazard lights in the background between sentences.[9]

I'd phoned him because he heads clinical practice at Carrier Sekani Family Services, an organization dedicated to bringing badly needed mental health care to Indigenous communities in northern BC that would otherwise have none. Their aim is prevention and ongoing treatment, but suicide attempts and suicidal ideation are their bread and butter. A couple of weeks before we spoke, he told me, he got four calls in one day from four different communities. In one case, they arrived too late. The year before they got a call from the RCMP about fourteen kids ("well, kids under thirty") who'd tried to kill themselves in one area in a single weekend.

"We were running around at night trying to find them and trying to stabilize. . . . Some people, their relatives had taken them to hospitals in a nearby town; some people were there; some people were hiding; some people were drinking in the bush. Everything. We had a team. We brought in, I think, six people that night. We went door to door and one at a time knocked them off the list."

Stabilizing these crises is about as bare-bones a triage as you can imagine. If the person is relatively low-risk (thinking about suicide but not concretely or imminently planning it), Poschwatta's team will make sure they have ongoing supports and leave them at home.

"If it turns into moderate risk, where there's a fairly detailed plan, and they haven't done anything and they don't really want to, but it's there, then we need 24/7 mature, sober people . . . doing shift work until we get enough mental health work in to reduce that risk down to minimal."

If there's no one sufficiently reliable on hand, "we get creative. . . . You know, 'Where's your cousins? Where's your uncles? Where's your grandma?' Well, in the next village there's an uncle and he's been sober for twenty-two years and we phone over and he's there and he's willing to take him in for a few days.

"This is not easy work."

Assessing the degree of danger a person poses to themselves in that moment is brutally tricky at the best of times, and Poschwatta's team has no specialized training in how to do it. That weighs heavily on him. "I don't know how many suicides I've assessed—well over a hundred, anyway. I would like to have that backup, have a hotline where there's experts available to review what I've heard." More often than not, it's just him and his colleagues making that judgment call—will this kid be safe here, on her own, with these people who love her but who may be struggling with problems of their own, who may not be able to babysit a young adult indefinitely? Will she survive the night? "If we don't have anyone there, then it's just take 'em to the hospital. By hook or by crook, get 'em to the hospital." He pauses. "But we find that's a problem."

You'd think taking someone in the grips of suicidality to the nearest hospital would at least get them through the crisis. Keep them safe until someone capable can figure out a plan of care. Not so much.

"All they do is ask people, 'Are you suicidal?' And if they say, 'No,' and there's no sign—like, they don't have rope burns around their neck or something—they let them go."

That can be a deadly mistake.

"We've had situations that went sideways. We worked our butts off and we thought they were in there and we thought we had a doctor onside, they were going to hold them for an assessment or whatever, and an hour later we get a phone call: they're back on the street. They lied to the doctor. They said, 'I'm okay, I don't need any help.' So we have to run around on the street and phone the cops again," Poschwatta says, aggravation in his voice. "We had seven in one year that suicided within one day of being in emergency. . . . If it was non-Aboriginal people I'm pretty sure there would be a stink to high heaven. There would be inquiries and god knows what."

And in the Lower Mainland, after Brian David Geisheimer and Sarah Louise Charles and Sebastien Pavit Abdi walked out of the psych ward and obliterated themselves, there was. That doesn't happen in the small, largely Indigenous communities in the same province a thousand kilometres away. The inquest-spurring outcry isn't there.

In Hazelton, a 270-person community in northwest BC, the staff at Carrier Sekani took matters into their own hands: they set up their own suicide crisis unit next door to the hospital and got clinicians with existing gigs elsewhere to commit time to staff it. Post-discharge suicides dropped almost immediately.

Once they've managed to get people stable, Poschwatta and his team sit them down in a group, make safety plans and start honing in on what's driving them to want to die. Some people need to talk one-on-one with a health worker; some feel better going over their triggers of despair with others who are experiencing the same kind of thing.

There's a lot of trauma: people who've been abused by parents, uncles, elders who were abused themselves. A lot of self-medication with alcohol. "It might be after two or three days working with them we decide this one needs to go to provincial alcohol and drug treatment, or this one needs a psych assessment. So we just keep working and listening until we come up with a plan for each person."

None of this is fun. "It's gruelling," he says. "I'm not happy about it. I wish it would go away. . . . It's not a job. It's like I'm here to do this to help them, 'cause nobody else will."

The proactive work's a bit less soul-destroying. The staff at Carrier Sekani have started focusing on depression screening for everyone. Apparently, the secret is not to mention the D-word while doing it. "We have some very nice people explain to the people that this is a little checkup that will let you know how you're doing in terms of mental health."

Also, bribery. People who get the checkup get free lanyards with their clan symbol on them and are entered in a draw for an iPad.

Then cultural liaisons go in and nudge the people who've been flagged toward treatment. "We're very gentle, like right off the bat it'd be, 'There are some things we'd like to talk to you about, would you be available to go for a cup of coffee or something like that?' And we try to steer them to services."

Ideally you'd get care where you live, or close to it. But it's tough convincing clinicians to move to communities of a few dozen or a couple of hundred people in the middle of temperate rainforest wilderness. Tougher still to get outside clinicians who can actually earn the trust of the people they're caring for.

"And then," Henry Harder tells me when I phone him in Prince George, a 75,000-person city in northern British Columbia, "there's the whole issue of stigma: if you're a community of a couple hundred people, the mental health therapist arrives in town and now you're lining up, everyone knows you're going. So . . . you tend to not go."[10]

I had called him to try and get my head around the gap in mental health care for Indigenous people. He figures he's one of ten psychologists in Prince George, which is also a service hub for dozens of remote communities.

He knows you won't get the best mental health care in every tiny community—but telepsychiatry is known to work, he says, if not as well as in-person visits at least much better than nothing, or the fumbling best efforts of someone who isn't well-versed in psychic pain. But telepsychiatry is grossly underutilized: only 1 percent of Ontarians who need psychiatric care get it through telepsychiatry, even in remote communities where that otherwise means going without any care at all for a year or more.[11] At least it can get you a diagnosis, an assessment outside of the nearest (distant) emergency department's frantic scrum. A prescription, maybe. Or an informed opinion, with perhaps a referral to an urban centre if you need specific services, one that will ensure you get those services once you arrive.

"We've got to do a good job of getting them assessed and getting them out and, for god's sake, helping them get back to their community. They're just dumped out the front door of their hospital."

Seriously.

He knows people who've been left penniless outside the Prince George hospital to fend for themselves in a city that isn't theirs because neither level of government will take responsibility for transporting them back to their home. The federal government is responsible for health care on-reserve and the provincial government is responsible for health care off-reserve and their tussles over whose job it is to transfer someone who travelled to the city to get care back to the reserve often leaves the person—often a kid—stranded.

"People fall through the cracks pretty easily," said Cindy Hardy, who is also a psychologist in Prince George and who I reached out to because of her work on the ways people fall through those cracks.[12] Health systems fail people in the most basic ways but also in the less obvious ones. Let's say you make an appointment to see a psychiatrist or psychologist in a big city a few hundred kilometres away. Jackpot—congratulations. Now you need to negotiate the time off work, arrange the child care, maybe figure out where you're going to spend the night if you can't make the six-hour drive there and back in one day. Maybe you have a car and can afford gas; maybe you get a voucher for the bus. Or maybe you can't swing the bus schedule so you're left hitching a ride on a highway that's become synonymous with missing and murdered Indigenous women. Good luck making that appointment. "If they don't show up for appointments or they don't call, they're off the list—that's it. So when you're feeling really depressed and you can't get out of bed, that's easy to do. They just fall off the radar."

Indigenous people are supposed to have extended health coverage. But, guess what: you need to make a special application for psychotherapy.

"Isn't that ridiculous?" she exclaims. "People are looking for help and they have to go through all these hoops. And I see this repeatedly with insurers. . . . The paperwork is more of a barrier if your literacy is low, or if you don't have access to a supportive physician." Annoying paperwork can be a barrier for therapists as much as patients: busy professionals would rather not spend time filling out forms. "Especially when we have a load of other people who don't require that much paperwork, yeah, we're going to go with the path of least resistance, right?"

(In case you were wondering, I did email the federal government's health department: How many requests for mental health care are made each year, and how many are granted, under Canada's health benefits program covering Indigenous people? But they refused to say.)

Media frenzies around clusters of Indigenous youth suicides—like the one when Jolynn and Chantell and Jenera killed themselves, like when a slew of young people in Attawapiskat First Nation killed themselves the year before—drive her Prince George colleague Henry Harder nuts.

"Indigenous suicide becomes some sort of a banner call for people, and words like 'epidemic' and 'crisis' get used." The feast-and-famine way news organizations cover Indigenous suicide makes it easier for politicians and policymakers to cast around for "a quick, hopefully easy and hopefully cheap solution to the problem."

"When the government freaks out and they send a whole bunch of clinicians into one area, that helps for a little while. But everybody piles back out again and everything goes back to where it was before," he says. "To me, the solution here is to provide adequate services and health care and food and opportunities into those communities long before they have a suicide issue. . . . If I could have a big banner it would say, 'Give that money beforehand.'" But all too often projects meant to bridge chasms end mid-air. "We seem to always go partway down a path and then the funding stops. The initiative stops. And it never fully develops." And even when there is funding for health interventions, the execution falls flat. You'll have half-a-dozen different pilot projects under different government umbrellas doing different things in a single place. "You could have one community approached by three or four different groups all coming to say, 'Well, we're here to help you with your suicide prevention.'" It doesn't really foster trust when you feel more like an anthropological experiment than a group of humans meriting the same care as your fellow citizens.

"This sounds like a bit of a broken record, but one of the things Canadian society struggles with over and over again is the whole issue of the residential school legacy. And a great deal of the mental illness issues, especially on reserve, lead directly back to that legacy.

And until we just stop pretending that never happened, or pretend like throwing money at it or making an apology in Ottawa is going to change that, then we're going to continue having these issues. We have to help communities deal with that. There are people who were sexually abused in their residential schools who are sexual abusers on reserve. And they are in leadership positions and kids tell me they can't go for help to the elders because they're abusing them.

"How do you break that cycle?"

"I make presentations all over the world," he says wearily, "and I get a better reception outside of Canada than I do in Canada. In Canada you get kind of some version of, 'Get over it.' I'm serious. It's like, 'That was a long time ago. Canada has apologized. We've given those Indians a hell of a lot of money. Why don't they just get over it?'"

MICHAEL KIRLEW—Jolynn, Chantell and Jenera's doctor—uses the phrase "transformation" a lot when he talks about what needs to happen to make Indigenous health care anything other than a cruel joke "structured to deny care." He believes the set-up, the people running it, the care that's provided and the way decisions are made, all need to be wholly transformed.[13] "Child mental health has to go from being considered a program to a right."

He sees young kids with developmental disabilities that never get treated because the federal government won't cover the cost of travel to a city with specialists capable of assessing their needs. He's had travel requests to see a doctor denied because a patient saw the doctor eight months earlier. So kids grow up lacking necessary care, struggling to cope at home and in school, where as students they receive less funding, per capita, than their non-Indigenous counterparts. If, like a huge proportion of Indigenous kids, they're in foster care, they can have been through dozens of homes by the time they hit puberty, which means that what care they get is truncated. "It becomes a recipe for disaster."

Worse than all this, though, is the way a system that undervalues you in the most literal way reinforces the suicidal sense that you don't matter.

"Colonization really works to take away your hope—hope in justice, hope in fairness, hope in health equity. . . . Youth might lose hope because of all the different things that have happened in their lives, because of all this trauma, but, as well, because they interface with a system that has told them that they are hopeless and they have no value."

What do you tell a suicidal twelve-year-old?

"I tell every single one of those youths that their life is valuable— that [their] life has purpose. . . . They may have never heard that before."

23

Race as Barrier

Mental illness is expert at compounding existing marginalizations—taking aspects of your life that make you vulnerable and using them to screw you further.

So it is with race. Not being white can make you not only less likely to get in the door to get care, but less likely to get good care and less likely to stick around long enough for that care to work. Things that might otherwise be protective—a close-knit community, family ties, a commitment to stoic strength—can work against you. Even the most basic need to be *seen* by the people providing your care can prove elusive, shafting your shot at help that makes a positive difference.

Let's be clear: I am not a person of colour and I don't live with the burdens, don't face the barriers that entails. I've tried to read as much and talk to as many people as I could to rectify my own innate ignorance, because frankly this barrier to adequate, effective mental health care—ranging from systemic racism to therapeutic incongruence—is too urgent, too deadly not to address head-on.

A 2010 National Institute of Mental Health study found that while only one-fifth of Americans with depression got the right kind of care for their condition, African Americans, Caribbean Black and Mexican Americans were half as likely to get good care.

And while health insurance may enable better access to depression care, it does not ensure better care.¹ Latinx Americans in need of mental health care are less likely to get it, less likely to see a specialist, more likely to experience delays and, when they do get care, less likely to get anything congruent with guidelines and less likely to be satisfied with the care they get.²

An American study of Medicaid enrollees found the most marginalized or seriously ill people were least likely to get minimally adequate care. Black people and those who began depression treatment with an inpatient psychiatric stay for depression were less likely to receive minimally adequate psychotherapy and more likely to receive inadequate treatment.³

When it comes to accessing health care, poverty and geography can screw you in terms of getting in the door; race can keep screwing you once you're there. There are insidious hurdles—a health practitioner treats you a certain way, makes assumptions about you and what you need, fails to see you for you because of the way you look. You're made to feel unwelcome, uncared for.

A nurse almost gave eighteen-year-old Rudayna Bahubeshi someone else's medication when she confused her with the only other Black woman in the mood disorder inpatient unit. She had been enveloped in a depressive vortex that yanked her out of her life, out of her final weeks of high school and into a psych hospital. What may seem like a minor, malice-less slip on the nurse's part made her feel shut out of an ostensibly universal health care system. "After several weeks of feeling increasingly hopeless in the hospital, I checked myself out. For many years, I didn't seek mental health support," she wrote in a 2017 opinion piece for the CBC. "I can't say those who were negligent in overseeing my care had malicious intentions or made conscious assumptions related to my identity. But at the end of the day, do intentions matter when the ways in which I was vulnerable were overlooked and unacknowledged?"⁴

Interventions won't work if you can't connect. Clinicians are trying to fix your brain, not your bike.

An effective therapist doesn't need to be their patient's demographic twin. They just need to be cognizant of what people different from them are going through.

The newbie psychologists Rheeda Walker advises look at her askance when she tells them to ask new patients about the role race and culture play in their lives. In their first session, even. In a written questionnaire, if they'd rather. It's key to understanding where a person is coming from, she tells me. And it's often something people won't bring up on their own, "because you don't want to make other people feel uncomfortable."[5] I'd called her up—a psychologist and head (and founder) of the University of Houston's Culture, Risk, and Resilience Lab—to help shed some light on psychological racial disparities. She speaks with the patient authority of an expert who breaks down her expertise to the clueless for a living. (Our phone conversation took place on November 9, 2016, the day after the US election, a day when much of the world was reeling and, she noted, a day when cultural sensitivity would be a must if you're a health practitioner.)

It's often tempting to hope that not mentioning race neutralizes it as an issue. But if race or cultural background is a key part of your identity, if it affects the way you experience the world and your own psychological pain, ignoring it can doom a therapeutic relationship. "So you can see how termination might happen prematurely. It's like, 'I don't even know why I'm talking to them. I should just go somewhere else.' Or they don't go anywhere."

Walker, who is Black, sees two barriers to access for African Americans: getting in the door, and sticking with treatment long enough to get well. The former is often influenced by a combination of socio-economic factors—we know poverty and isolation discriminate along stark racial lines—and the assumption you don't need or deserve help.

The tendency of Black Americans and other minorities to quit care is complex but it's attributable in part to a sense of un-belonging, Walker says. And it's on the clinician to address it. "There's this idea that, 'Oh, no one's even presenting themselves for care.' And I think, no, the burden is on the therapist that when someone does show up, you make an extra effort to keep that person in care. Even if you're uncomfortable."

Gursharan Virdee, who is a Toronto-based psychologist and researcher, tells me she sees it in the patients she works with—young South Asian Canadian women who come to her multilingual practice after seeking mental health help from more mainstream providers and not feeling seen.

"I've worked with a young woman who wears hijab, was never asked by her therapist about her religion and so on, and the not asking actually led this young woman to disengage because she didn't feel empowered to share or kind of talk from that position," she says to me by phone.[6] Another young woman felt her former therapist didn't get her family dynamic, where she was undervalued relative to the men in her family and how that factored into pathological feelings of worthlessness. "There's a lack of awareness of the role of culture in one's experience and how that might shape a person's mental health."

Napoleon Harrington, a Michigan-based counsellor who focuses much of his work and advocacy on communities of colour, sees three factors preventing Black Americans from accessing mental health care when they need it. One is a cultural mythology of strength. "We've been identified as a strong people, and when strength is mischaracterized it gets identified as not needing support or not needing help or not being willing to depend on resources that may in one regard oppress you and maybe in another way render you weak. So I think because strength has been mischaracterized in our culture it gives the impression that we can't find those resources."[7]

The second is religion—a powerful protective factor when it comes to thinking of killing yourself, but also a potential deterrent from seeking secular care. "Reliance on God is extremely heavy, and reliance on God to cure you, to deliver you, to heal you and all of those conversations that come from each of those convictions . . . [means] I don't have faith if I get help."

The third: Would you trust your thoughts and feelings to a doctor, a counsellor, embedded within a system with a long history of treating you and people who look like you like lesser persons? "Black folks and brown folks have a challenge with a system that has not always been in their best interest . . . it makes us very, very mistrusting of anybody who works within that system." And if people of colour are more likely to be incarcerated and more likely to have their kids taken from them by child welfare agencies, maybe you're less likely to confide in a clinician with the power to set either of those things in motion.

Of those three factors, Harrington is best positioned to tackle the first—to convince people of colour, especially in the Black community, that mental health is something that should be on their mind, that mental health care is something they may need and that there's no shame in seeking it. He tries to meet people where they're at; use straightforward "stigma-free" language; use slang and Ebonics if it seems helpful.

I ask him, a Black counsellor, if he has advice for a white clinician working with people of colour. What should they take into account, without projecting?

"The intolerant history of America and its behaviour toward Black and brown people has created a layer of anxiety, trauma, depression, you name it . . . a layer that's palpable enough for anyone who's brown in America to feel it. . . . So I think the major difference is, every time you're working with someone of a Black or brown context, [remember that] that layer somehow is always present even if they're wildly successful, they have enough money or what have you, they will always meet something or someone that reminds them that race is still present."

JASMIN

No one thought to ask Jasmin what was going on in her mind when she tried to annihilate herself. When she swallowed a pack of high-strength allergy medication and wound up delirious and hospitalized. Not when her mom came to the emergency department to meet her and the panicked friends who'd rushed her there. Not when she drank, at nurses' urging, an activated charcoal smoothie to keep toxins from sinking into her system. Not when she was discharged back out into the world.

"Why didn't anyone think to say, 'Are you depressed? What's going on?' I just knew I wanted to die."[8]

Eighteen years old, getting over a bad breakup, preparing to move out of her mom's place and go to college, Jasmin felt her life become inexplicably unbearable. "I just felt like the walls were closing in on me."

That time—the first time—the decision to swallow the entire off-brand allergy prescription she'd just filled was entirely impulsive. "I wasn't really thinking straight. . . . After I did it, I was like, 'Why did I do that?' I didn't understand."

In the hospital, with her worried mom and friends, Jasmin felt more embarrassed than anything. They asked, "'Why would you do something like that? Why would you want to take your own life?' I told them there was a lot going on."

She was mad at herself. She felt stupid. Overemotional, over-reacting. "After a while I just let it go."

And that was that. Jasmin moved from Kentucky to Louisiana, living with her dad in New Orleans while she went to college.

But it didn't go well and she didn't know why. She couldn't concentrate, kept having to retake classes. Kept messing up orders at the pizza place where she worked. She blamed her skittering brain on distractedness. Admonished herself to do better.

But the walls kept closing in. The second time, at age twenty, Jasmin meant it. "The second time I was like, 'Okay, I know for sure I don't want to be here anymore.'"

She swallowed a bottle of Tylenol. Her dad, home from work early, found her and took her to hospital. This time it took a tube snaking down her throat to exhume the poison. Thirty minutes watching gunk slurp through the clear plastic tube clawing against her esophagus.

"That was a really horrible day. . . . I was mad that it didn't work."

This time, she was sent to a psychiatric facility. "It was a really nice place, but of course I didn't want to be there. I didn't want anybody to be all up in my business." And it freaked her out to be in close quarters for the first time with people with severe mental illness, behaving erratically. She wasn't one of them, she told herself. She wasn't nuts. "It was scary. I saw things I'd never seen before. . . . At the time I was like, 'Why do you have me in here with people like this?' I was angry. I wanted to leave. . . . My family came and saw me a few times. I felt so embarrassed: here she is, in a psychiatric hospital."

She refused to talk to the psychiatrist at first, furious at her captivity. Changed tack the second day "because I was determined to get out of there and I knew if I didn't talk to anybody, I couldn't."

He diagnosed her with depression. The diagnosis was not comforting.

"It actually felt worse. I just thought that people who had mental illness were crazy. That's what you saw on TV," she said. "I'm like, 'Well, I'm not crazy, so why are they telling me I'm depressed?'"

For six months Jasmin got what vanishingly few depressed people get: evidence-based treatment. Antidepressants *and* psychotherapy based on science. Unfortunately, six months is a nanosecond when it comes to chronic mood disorders. The meds dampened her depression but didn't alleviate it. When the side effects—irritability and insomnia were the worst—threatened to eclipse the symptoms the drugs tried to treat, she went off them entirely. "You get really frustrated after a while." Her psychiatric visits lasted a few months more. "He was a good doctor, but I still wasn't really comfortable talking about my feelings or emotions." In a lot of ways, Jasmin knows, she was still in denial. Refused to consider herself crazy. Didn't tell anyone for fear they'd respond the same way she had when confronted with her fellow psych patients.

Community support systems can be a powerful protective factor for anyone dealing with mental illness, but she discovered that deep-seated communal misconceptions about sicknesses of the brain can make them worse.

"I think that one of the reasons I was so in denial for so long and I thought people with mental illness were crazy was because in the Black community, they make you think you're just supposed to pray away a mental illness. It's like, 'Oh, you're depressed? Well you're not praying enough. You need to get closer to God.' I think that's the worst thing to tell somebody: How do you know someone with a mental illness hasn't already been praying? How do you know they're not close to God? Telling somebody something like that, it makes them feel worse."

Jasmin's still trying to figure out what it is that makes her community's exhortations to stick-to-itiveness backfire when it comes to psychological resilience, why it remains so tough to reconcile the capacity to survive waves of collective and personal trauma with the reality that overwhelming psychic pain comes in different, uncontrollable forms.

"I think it goes back generations. A lot of Black people feel like we got through slavery, we got through all this, we're supposed to be strong all the time. But don't you think they were depressed back then? Just because you got through something doesn't mean you don't still have emotions."

Even Jasmin's dad, who never judged, who wanted to help, who wanted to convince his daughter her life was worth living, made things tougher sometimes. "There were times when he was like, 'You need to be stronger than this.' He never told me to snap out of it, but he's like, 'You have a lot going for yourself.' That's not a really good thing to tell someone who has a mental illness. But he didn't understand that at the time."

Then there was the worst year. Jasmin was out of school, out of treatment and shortly out of a job. That last, especially, was a body blow. "I'd never been fired from a job in my life. The walls were

closing in on me again. This was years of everything finally building up." She overdosed on every drug she could lay her hands on.
Prescription and off the pharmacy shelf and everything at the back
of the medicine cabinet. Benadryl, Tylenol, high-strength nasal
decongestant, "four different prescription medications all at once."

The nurses saved her life and Jasmin was miserable about it. "I was
like, 'I took all of this medication and I'm still alive?' I felt like a failure.
'I fail at life and I fail at trying to kill myself. This is just ridiculous.'"

Jasmin spent almost a week in intensive care before being transferred to a different psychiatric inpatient facility, this one a couple
of hours out of town.

When she assured them she had a psychiatrist already (the guy
she'd stopped seeing a while back), they discharged her relatively
quickly. Her twenty-sixth birthday was the following week.

It was not a great birthday. By that point she really, really, really
needed to get better. She could not countenance another trip to
the ICU, another psychiatric sojourn, that claustrophobic sense of
failure.

Then she found psychic respite in the unlikeliest confidante: a
friend of her dad's with no formal training but who listened in a way
no one else did. "I finally found someone I can talk to and feel good
afterward. . . . It's hard to find someone who'll actually listen to you."
And she started doing research. It was revelatory.

"I thought I was alone the whole time. I never knew that many
people, millions of people, suffer from it every day. . . . It's like a
silent illness no one wants to talk about."

She worked up the courage to tell people. Friends and family at
first. Then everyone who would listen. She made a video of her
experience, posted it on YouTube.

"I was really afraid to make that video. I made it one time and I
deleted it and then I made it again. It took a couple of weeks to actually post it." Was taken aback at the positive response. "'You look
fine on the outside but on the inside you're not okay.' That's the kind
of response."

So she kept talking. Wrote a book. Participated in a documentary that screened at the Tribeca Film Festival.

It's a redemptive story even if she knows it isn't over. Remission isn't the same as cure. Recovery doesn't preclude relapse. But "I'm not ashamed of it anymore. . . . I wanted other people to realize they're not crazy, either."

IF RACE CAN be a barrier, so can culture. Reluctance to seek treatment for a progressively debilitating chronic illness—because you don't think you need it or deserve it or the shame associated with seeking a cure seems worse than anything illness can throw at you—means that by the time you get necessary care, the disorder's already had a chance to rip your guts out.

Maria Chiu, staff scientist with the not-for-profit Institute for Clinical Evaluative Sciences (ICES) in Toronto, has seen that reticence play out along ethnic and cultural lines: South Asian Canadian and Chinese Canadian patients admitted to a psychiatric emergency department in a Toronto hospital were in much more acute condition when they arrived compared with others in the psych ER with them. Chiu's research revealed that Chinese patients were more likely to be admitted against their will, were more likely to be acting aggressively and were more likely to have more than three symptoms of a serious illness. South Asian patients were also more likely to be showing signs of a severe mental illness compared with the general population.[9] This held true across the board. "We controlled for everything—age, sex, income, education, immigration status, marital status, urban or rural residents," she says. "As well as the diagnosis, which is really important. I can't think of anything else we could have adjusted for, because we took into account a lot."[10]

Culture can mediate both what a person considers a mental illness and how comfortable they feel getting help for it. Fear of what seeking medical help for your mind says about you, fear of what your family or friends or community will think of you, shame at having this problem keep you from seeking help even if you're pretty sure something is not right. There may be more reluctance to share these shameful conditions with outsiders.

"You don't want to bring shame to the family either. And if people feel like, 'Oh, that's the family of the person who's mentally ill—avoid them at all costs,'" Chiu says. "Then it's also hard to find a job, it's hard to find a husband or a wife in certain cultures."

Or people view this as something to be dealt with discreetly at home, in private. "Mental hospitals in general have a bad rap. You think, 'I don't want to be a psych patient: people will think I'm crazy.'" So they try to manage on their own until they can't, and they end up in hospital whether they want to be there or not. Even in families or communities that have been in Canada for generations, Chiu says, there remains an ethos that "we have to work really hard for what we have, we should not show weakness—these are things that you're taught very young, especially if you're an ethnic minority. And so having mental illness is seen as a weakness."

A lack of language facility or knowledge of the health system can act as systemic barriers to accessing care too. That's something you'd expect to see with relatively recent immigrants, but the study's findings held true whether someone was a recent immigrant, had arrived in the country more than a decade earlier, or had been born and lived their entire lives there. "It's the ethnicity or the culture that seems to be more important than the immigration status. . . . You may not be as willing to share your story or your struggle because you may not think your provider can relate," Chiu says.

We know that catching mental illness early can prevent it from getting worse, can make it less likely to recur. The immediate and long-term harms of not addressing serious health problems early are obvious. So is the irony: by delaying care because the idea of a mental illness is too freaky to contemplate, people deteriorate and end up receiving that care in the freakiest manner possible. It affects the health care system, because hospitalization is the most costly and intensive treatment option out there.

And the response to Chiu's research paper, once it was published, is enough to indicate she's onto something. "People shared stories," she tells me, "saying, 'I've been through something similar; it was hard to talk to my family.' It's been really, really eye-opening, and really gratifying that it reached a wide audience."

Her follow-up study had more encouraging findings: even though they show up in hospital in worse mental shape, Chinese and South Asian Canadians got better once they connected with care. Chinese patients were more likely to see psychiatrists; South Asian patients were more likely to seek mental health care from general practitioners; both were less likely to die or wind up back in hospital in the year following their hospitalization.[11]

Sometimes the way you've grown up, the community you're in, can preclude even conceptualizing a mood disorder. Clinical depression "simply did not exist within the realm of my possibilities; or, for that matter, within the realm of possibilities for any of the black women in my world," Meri Nana-Ama Danquah writes in her book *Willow Weep for Me: A Black Woman's Journey through Depression.* Danquah, born in Ghana and raised in the US, is a writer, editor and public speaker. "The one myth that I have had to endure my entire life is that of my supposed birthright to strength. Black women are *supposed* to be strong—caretakers, nurturers, healers of other people—any of the twelve dozen variations of Mammy. Emotional hardship is *supposed* to be built into the structure of our lives. It went along with the territory. . . . When a black woman suffers from a mental disorder, the overwhelming opinion is that she is weak. And weakness in black women is intolerable. I've frequently been told things like: 'Girl, you've been hanging out with too many white folk'; 'What do you have to be depressed about? If our people could make it through slavery, we can make it through anything'; 'Take your troubles to Jesus, not no damn psychiatrist.'"

Danquah recalls the sense of disoriented invalidation she got from her white male psychiatrist.

"Phew," she remembers him saying after she told him about being treated like a thief when returning a dress in a clothing store—an act of "everyday racism" all the more galling for its banality. "It must be so hard to be black. I can't even fathom having to contend with what you must deal with on a daily basis." A well-meaning, honest statement, sure. But that inability to fathom someone else's experience makes therapeutic congruence just about impossible.

"I do not believe that white therapists are unable to successfully treat people of colour," Danquah writes. "However, I do think that they should possess a certain level of cultural sensitivity, as that culture plays an important role in both the patient's illness and treatment. I am black; I am female; I am an immigrant. Every one of these labels plays an equally significant part in my perception of myself and the world around me."[12]

PART IV

IN THE MAZE

24

Who You Gonna Call?

Police are the wrong people to call when someone's suicidal, says Susan Stefan, an author and expert on psychiatric disabilities and the law. I called her to get a better sense of the interplay of rights, legalities and first-responder imperatives when dealing with people in crisis.

"You'll see people who call the police and they'll say, 'I want to commit suicide by cop; send the police.' . . . And what do they do? They send over eight armed police officers."

"You're joking."

"No, I'm not joking. And guess what happens. . . . When you're in psychiatric crisis almost anything is better than calling 911."[1]

I know plenty of people who would dispute that. But whether it's the best option or not, psych crisis calls make up a growing proportion of cops' workload.

Calling first responders or having first responders called on you when you're in crisis is fundamentally about a loss of control: they're there to take charge; you're calling them because you want them to take charge. I've talked to people who found it reassuring—that's the point of calling 911—but it engenders a panicky desperation when the thing they're saving you from is yourself.

I've been lucky in my interactions with police and paramedics but I suspect it's in part because I'm a short white girl and I was cowed

and obedient. I don't know what would have happened if I'd struggled or yelled or talked back when I was ordered into the back of a
cop car or ambulance. Or what would have happened if I was a male
of colour—in Toronto, the city where I was picked up, Black people
made up 60 percent of fatal interactions with police despite only
comprising 8.8 percent of the population.[2]

When people call 911, they do so assuming that those whose
job it is to serve and protect them will serve and protect them in
one of the most vulnerable points of their lives. But, too often, disclosure can ostracize, can disqualify. Calling for help can make you
regret it and making people regret calling for help means they won't
seek it again when they desperately need it.

In Halifax, mental illness–related calls doubled between 2007
and 2014; Calgary's "Million-Dollar Martin," a sick man who cost
the city about $1 million in cop calls within a year, has achieved
urban-legend status among harm-reduction acolytes.[3] The recently
retired head of Toronto's civilian police watchdog has suggested the
prevalence of mental illness in officers' day-to-day jobs necessitates
not just changes in training, but radically different recruitment
strategies—hiring officers with empathy, who won't freak out or
revert to prejudicial stereotypes when they encounter people struggling with psychiatric maladies. Maybe even giving preference to
those with some psychology training.[4]

But often, things get ugly. Sometimes, you get tasered. In dozens
of cases over an eighteen-month period in Canada's largest city,
Toronto police tasered mentally unstable, suicidal people who posed
no threat to anyone but themselves. More than half of all Taser uses
in 2014 were on "emotionally disturbed persons," according to cops'
own reporting. About a third of those people were apprehended
under Ontario's Mental Health Act. Officers believe the people
they're confronting are armed 60 percent of the time, when in reality only about a third (in Toronto) are bearing anything that could
be used as a weapon.

Tasers are fired more often in the west-end neighbourhood of

Parkdale, where I used to live, which has a higher proportion of people with mental illness than any other area of the city. I wrote about this in an article for Global News: "Police tasered a suicidal man twice—once in the stomach and once in the back—'to gain compliance' as he resisted being apprehended and handcuffed by officers. In one instance, an officer tried to taser a man cutting his throat with a knife, but missed as the suicidal man backed toward his balcony. The rest of the incident report is censored: it isn't clear whether the man killed himself. . . . On multiple occasions, the suspect was tasered after already being forced to the ground by police. One man with mental illness, believed to be both drunk and high, was tasered three times while held on the ground by police. Another was tasered multiple times while lying on a mattress where he was apprehended."[5] Tasers are marketed as a "non-lethal" weapon and much of the public discourse around their use assumes they're used when an officer might otherwise use a gun. That isn't how it works. Conducted energy weapons aren't as reliable as firearms: if you really needed the latter, you wouldn't use the former. Tasers are a step or so down the use-of-force scale and officers use them when someone is acting violently or erratically or is resisting in some way when they're trying to restrain them or when they have already been restrained. "My opinion is that if you really use Tasers at times when you would have otherwise used a firearm, then they're great: I'd rather be tased than shot," says Joel Dvoskin, a forensic psychologist who's designed psychiatric hospitals and trained people in dealing with psych crises, whom I reach by phone. "But the problem is that a lot of departments, once they start using Tasers, their use of Tasers is way higher than their use of lethal force was before. Because it's easier."[6]

We still don't really know what the health effects of a Taser are because the people most likely to be tasered are the least healthy and therefore the least likely to be included in any study and the most complex for divining a single cause of death. People have died after or shortly after being hit with these weapons but causation is tricky to determine. A Reuters investigation found more than 150 autopsy reports citing Tasers as a contributing factor in a person's death; frequently, those people were unarmed and in psychological distress.[7] In many cases where someone who is drunk or high or in the grips of severe mental illness dies after being tasered, their death is attributed to "excited delirium," a medical condition not recognized by most medical associations but which keeps coming up at inquests.

Whether incapacitating a suicidal someone with a painful electric shock is a good idea depends on whom you ask. You may be saving their life. You may be doing nothing of the sort, if they stumble and fall off the roof they've been threatening to jump off or if they seize and slit their throat with the knife they've been threatening to slit their throat with. Or, more likely, in my view, you just ensure they will never call the police or tell anyone they're feeling suicidal ever again.

"People say it's inhumane" to taser people who only pose a danger to themselves, says Memphis Police Lt. Colonel Vincent Beasley, who coordinates the force's pioneering Crisis Intervention Team and who talked to me by phone. "Is it really inhumane, or is it inhumane for me to sit there and watch you blow your brains out?"[8]

Beasley knows what he'd pick. And it isn't watching someone die by their own hand.

Who should get to know about your mental illness–related run-in with the cops? For a while, the guards at the Canada-US border would know—and they were refusing people entry to the United States because of their one-time suicidality. After much scrutiny and criticism—and the threat of a lawsuit from Ontario's privacy commissioner—Toronto Police agreed to block US Customs and Border Protection officers from seeing entries in Canada's police database. But they still enter every suicide-related call in there.[9]

Joel Dvoskin argues there's efficacy in information-sharing when it comes to people in psychological distress—but that it's important to keep the sharing circle tight. "If I'm a resident evaluating somebody in an emergency department 'cause somebody said they were suicidal and they say, 'Yeah, you know, I was just mad at my mother;

I'm not going to kill myself. Everything's fine,' but I look in the database and I see he tried to grab a police officer's gun a few days ago and the police officer cut him a break and didn't arrest him, now all of a sudden that's going to change my evaluation."

What are the alternatives to calling the cops? Susan Stefan points to Massachusetts' community crisis model as one to emulate because when someone's suicidal, social workers and mental health practitioners show up at your door, rather than cops. Massachusetts, with its 24/7 community psychiatric crisis teams, "is basically the Valhalla of the United States, in terms of social services"—even if there, too, you've only got so many crisis teams. The state has centres with designated crisis beds meant as an alternative to a trip to the ER and its hours-long wait in noisy fluorescent corridors for a psych assessment. But ambulances rarely take you there, she says. Instead those beds are often used as a "step-down" program for people after they're discharged.

She is also a fan of "recovery learning centres," peer-run support centres where you can go in and talk with no fear of anyone freaking out at your suicidality and committing you. For a contagion-theory proponent this is a terrifying prospect: people who all want to die *talking to each other about wanting to die?* Perhaps it calls to mind the online message boards of people trading suicide methods. But she assures me this isn't a room of people egging each other on to self-obliteration. "Most people feel tremendously alone and isolated and unable to talk about what they're going through and there's a real benefit of saying, 'Oh my god, I am not alone. I am not super-crazy.'"

CALLING THE POLICE when you're losing your mental or emotional shit doesn't have to be a nightmarish ordeal. The most oft-cited model is the Crisis Intervention Team.

Pioneered in Memphis, the Crisis Intervention Team model was propelled into being by a wrenching act of violence: in September 1987, Memphis police shot Joseph Robinson to death.

The twenty-seven-year-old Black man was stabbing himself with a knife; his mother had called police because she feared her son was suicidal. In the furor following his death at the cops' hands, a task force was created—which is hardly unusual. But this task force created something worthwhile that's being replicated in thousands of jurisdictions across the continent.

So far it's the gold standard: forty hours of training in dealing with people in the grips of mental illness, plus an additional eight every year.

It gets results. Lt. Colonel Vincent Beasley tells me that in the three decades since their CIT model was put in place, officer injuries from interactions with mentally ill individuals dropped 90 percent; civilian injuries dropped 75 percent. About 3.4 percent of the 18,435 mental illness calls Memphis police got in 2016 resulted in arrests (that's still more than 600 sick people being taken to penal facilities, though). About 30 percent of those interactions resulted in the person being taken to a health facility, such as a hospital; most of the time, officers are able to de-escalate the situation and, hopefully, address what precipitated it—by letting a person vent, by buying them a hamburger or a cigarette, by teaching their family how to cope—without carting someone off to an institution.

About a quarter of the Memphis police officers responding to calls have CIT training. There's at least one officer in each precinct at all times. It's key for them to be the first on the scene, he says. "The first few minutes of any situation are probably the most important ones. So if I get an officer there who doesn't understand this person is suffering from mental illness, they can do tons of damage before I get there." In many jurisdictions, they're only called in after conventional officers arrive and assess the situation. Or they're only available during certain times of day, or there's only one crisis intervention team for an entire city.

He got crisis intervention training a quarter-century ago because he saw firsthand the skills he was missing.

"In the area I worked in there were quite a few people who were suffering from mental illnesses. And I'm thinking, 'Hey, I'm answering these calls anyway. Why don't I learn about this so I can better serve those individuals?'"

What did he learn about people on the brink of suicide?

"They're fragile. And they want to commit suicide, but they don't want to commit suicide. . . . We just want the opportunity to talk to them."

The need for this training was driven home when Beasley's nephew Jacques killed himself. He was twenty-four. "He was a grandmama's boy, and just a great kid. Really. And I'm not just saying that. When he was five years old he memorized every page of a forty-eight-page book on Dr. Martin Luther King. And he went to every kindergarten school in the city of Memphis on a little circuit because they could not believe it."

But when Jacques was in college the grandmother who helped raise him died. And things began to fall apart. "I noticed it, but I didn't notice it," Beasley says. He asked his nephew if everything was okay and when Jacques said yes, he didn't press it.

"He taught me a lesson: to not take no for an answer. . . . I saw some of the same things in him that I saw in other people who were suffering from mental illnesses. But I didn't want to see that, because that was my nephew."

Just about every urban police force in North America will probably claim to have implemented or glanced at the CIT's principles to some degree. But there's tremendous variation in how good or effective or compassionate they are. A few years ago I visited a Toronto Police training centre and watched a de-escalation role play in which officers armed with Tasers talked down a man sitting at a table with a knife, threatening to kill himself. In that dramatized scenario, they were successful: he surrendered the plastic knife and they exited the mock apartment. The centre's classrooms were festooned with handwritten instructions on how to talk someone down: speak softly; ask non-aggressive questions; repeat what people have said back to them in a validating way.

But this is also a police force that tasered a woman *after* she dropped the knife she'd been holding to her throat; that shot to death a mentally ill man with a hammer within 120 seconds of entering the apartment hallway where he was standing. Who shot to death a man in a hospital gown holding scissors in the middle of a street. In moments of crisis, people don't always act in the way they would in a training module. When I spoke with Toronto police officers in charge of the frontline teams dealing with the mentally ill they noted that, of the thousands of interactions they have with people in crisis, the overwhelming majority go well.[10] And they're right. Or, at least, most interactions don't end in death.

But is that good enough? Alok Mukherjee doesn't think so. The former chair of Toronto's Police Services Board has argued for cop recruitment that focuses on compassion, on individuals' ability to work with people who are different from them; on "more people who say they're coming into policing because they want to help people, fewer who say they are here to catch the bad guys."

Crisis intervention trains officers to go slow. But "police officers are trained to go fast, not slow," Joel Dvoskin, the forensic psychologist, points out. "All the things police are trained to do—speak in a commanding voice; don't ask questions, give commands—none of that helps when a person's suicidal. So they have to kind of unlearn some things."

He figures there are two factors in the most acute suicide-prevention situations: options and time. If suicide is an escape from intolerable pain, finding an alternative escape, even a shallow transient one, can help. And stall. Stall for time in the hopes the most violent self-destructive impulse will attenuate just slightly.

"[If] you can keep them alive for a while, sometimes their natural defences kick in, they start thinking of other solutions," Dvoskin says. If nobody dies, then you win.

25

How to Talk about What We Talk about When We Talk about Wanting to Die

Imagine trying to cure cancer, or find an AIDS vaccine, or end world hunger or forcible human displacement, without ever mentioning the thing you're tackling. For ages that's been our approach to suicide, to the point that even the people paid to prevent it are loath to say its name.

Decades have conditioned us to avoid talking to someone about wanting to kill themselves, lest it seem like the act of discussing it is encouraging that act.

For many people, professionals and laypersons alike, the instinct is to dissuade—to plead, implore, exhort, *Don't do that!* And that's a legitimate response. And some people will want to hear that, or will at least take comfort in knowing people care about them and want them to live. "I'm glad you're alive" or "The world is better with you in it" are, I would argue, better ways of phrasing "Enough with this suicide!" But if your first response to someone's suicide attempt or their confession to wanting to die, is to say, "That's bad!" it can ensure that person never brings it up with you or anyone else ever again. No one wants to be lectured on the shittiness of their desires, no matter how self-destructive. "Family members will do that all day long. . . . Families are families. But clinicians, clinicians should be different than families," says David Jobes, a psychologist at the Catholic University of America. "Don't kill yourself!" is a valid emotional response to someone you care about. Clinician responses are not supposed to be fear- or emotion-driven. "You don't talk about the weather. You talk about, you know, you're here for a reason, and that reason is about life and death, and let's look at that."[1]

Crappy as we are at figuring out who has killed themselves, we're far worse at figuring out who's in danger of doing so. Much as I loathed being locked up against my will, I understand the excruciating nature of that calculation: Is she about to prance out of here and off herself? A 2016 study found clinicians evaluating suicide attempts in Winnipeg emergency rooms were laughably bad at guessing who was going to try again. Experience helped. Standardized assessment tools didn't.

Clinicians who went with their guts were 10 percent more likely to accurately predict a subsequent suicide attempt than clinicians who used a fancy-pants scale. People with more psychiatric experience were better at estimating reattempt risk. But not by much.[2]

Yunqiao Wang, one of the study's co-authors, expected accuracy rates to be low. As a psychologist with a practice of her own, she's seen how challenging risk assessment is. But she didn't expect them to be that low, she tells me by phone.[3] She knows the horror stories of people who kill themselves within twenty-four hours of discharge. Keeping them just a bit longer, to assess them a bit more thoroughly, might make a difference. "It's not enough to just, you know, 'Check, check, check, you meet the criteria' and then you're released."

Further complicating the prognostication game are people who "use suicide almost as a gesture"—a dramatic cry for help. There were a few people like that in the psych-ward rooms beside mine. Some had checked themselves in because they needed a respite from the responsibility of staying alive. Others, especially in the longer-term ward, cycled through repeatedly because they had nowhere else or nowhere better to go. Wang can understand this perspective but it irks her. "Crisis intervention is not a hotel."

Aaron Beck, one of America's most prominent psychiatrists and the father of cognitive therapy, formalized suicide risk factors into a scorecard: the seriousness of your attempt (Did you really think it would kill you? Did you really want it to?), the degree of premeditation (Did you put your affairs in order? Did you leave a note?), and the degree to which you tried to keep anyone from intervening (Were you alone, did you lock the door, did you wait for a moment when no one would notice your absence? Did you tell anyone?).[4] "It's a really complicated set of variables you have to factor in. But still, you're not going to be 100 percent right," says Paul Kurdyak at CAMH.[5]

Trust him: he's been there. One patient, in her mid-thirties or early forties, told him everything he needed to make him feel he could let her go. So he did. And she killed herself within hours. "Thankfully it's incredibly rare. But it is devastating." It can be brutal for staff psychiatrists to make discharge decisions knowing both how unreliable and how potentially deadly their best judgment is. "That's why I have a deep sense of humility about the task at hand."

When the Toronto family doctor Javed Alloo faces the challenge of sussing out a suicidal patient's likelihood of obliterating themselves before their next appointment, he'll ask if they're planning on killing themselves but knows that isn't enough on its own. "If they have interests and if they're feeling engaged with life, with hope of any kind, then I feel safer."[6] And he'll look at non-verbal cues— obvious ones, like the consistency of their answers, and ones that would never occur to me: Which way are their feet pointing? Are they responding to questions in a way that's different from the way they would normally respond?

One of his longtime patients with a history of chronic, near-debilitating non-mental illness ended up in emerg after overdosing on her medication, and he knew she was bullshitting when she told emergency staff it was an accident. "I'm like, no, she did it on purpose. Because she's not the type of person who makes mistakes." The next time she was sitting across from him in his office, he didn't mess around.

"'So, why'd you do it?' It was a purposely provocative question. She kind of looked at me and started to get ready a glib answer. And I just said, 'I know. So just tell me why you did it.' And then she told me. She told me, 'So I wouldn't be sad.'"

So he started her on depression treatment, and she stuck with it. His bold query made their doctor-patient relationship more open. "I felt more scared not asking the question than asking the question."

Of course it would be easier if there were a biomarker or a neurological test you could give someone to figure out how likely they are to try and kill themselves at some point in the future. "In cardiology," the National Institute of Mental Health's Sarah Lisanby points out, "we have EKGs, we have stress tests, we have ways of knowing if you are likely to die from your heart disease. We need the same for brain diseases. We need the same to know that this person in front of us, who is suffering from depression, is actually dying of it, is on their way to a future suicide."[7]

It sounds fanciful to me, or at least far away. But Maria Oquendo, past president of the American Psychiatric Association, does think it's possible. Some people who attempt suicide, she says, produce inordinate amounts of the hormone cortisol when they're stressed, and you can test for that in saliva. But even if you could disaggregate normal cortisol stress responses—if you're late for something or unprepared or otherwise stressed out—from super-high ones, that test wouldn't capture everyone. Some people's desire to die may be tied to abnormal serotonin systems and weirdnesses around receptor density. That's cumbersome to test for now, but she's confident that in a decade, that will change.[8]

Meanwhile, a group of researchers announced in 2017 that they'd designed a machine-learning algorithm that would read neural signatures of people's fMRIs, which measure brain activity by tracking changes in your blood flow. This could differentiate not only people thinking of suicide from people who aren't but people who'd attempted suicide from those who were just thinking about it.[9] This sounds futuristic and super-cool, but as someone whose liberty would likely be compromised by such a device, I'm leery. Apart from anything else, this still wouldn't tell you who is imminently going to try to kill themselves compared to those who just think about it all the time. If it worked it would no doubt flag me based on past actions and current ideation—but I'm not about to kill myself right now and I would absolutely object to being forcibly hospitalized as a result of such a scan.

We know more about what works and what doesn't work when it comes to treating people who want to die. It mostly involves talking to people about why they want to die and trying to help them deal with those things in a way other than death. That may sound obvious but it's a dramatic departure from the way clinicians—and just about everyone else—approach suicidality now.

"Typically, suicide is something that makes everybody uncomfortable, including clinicians," says Tom Ellis, the former senior staff psychologist at the Menninger Clinic. "So there's a really strong emotional pull on both parties' part to change the subject: 'Let's talk about your family; let's talk about your job; let's talk about various aspects of your life; but get off this business of wanting to die.'"[10] That strategy's not super efficacious. So he seeks to attack suicidality directly. "Let's prioritize, first and foremost, helping this person to survive." To do that, "we really need to understand what is beyond the disorder." He sits with patients and writes down what fuels their hopelessness and desire to die. "So it's very, very concrete, and very explicit."

People often know what their triggers are, but either way the therapist will talk things through with them, maybe suggesting things they aren't verbalizing even to themselves quite yet. He then develops a written safety plan with them "that says, you know, 'Let's see: What are your typical warning signs that you're about to go into a suicidal crisis? What sort of things have you learned in therapy that you can apply?'"

But the evidence suggests that a short-term intervention won't keep a chronic illness at bay for long. It's not enough to make someone feel life is worth living for a week or so, only to have them try and kill themselves a few months later, as several people in both the test and control groups did in a study Tom Ellis conducted. I've talked to people who felt way worse descending into despondency after a period of non-shittiness, because being reminded of the delta between hope and despair makes the latter that much more acute, the desperation to escape it that much more pressing.

Thing is, Catholic University of America psychology professor Dave Jobes says, you don't need that intensive inpatient environment. He designed a treatment model he calls Collaborative Assessment and Management of Suicidality that can be used in non-specialist outpatient settings—like your GP's office. He argues that talking directly to patients about the reasons behind their desire to die would save health systems a massive amount of money. "We call it sharpening the driver. . . . We ask the patient, 'What are the things that make you feel like you should take your life?'"

But asking if someone is thinking of killing themselves isn't enough if you ask the question the wrong way.

Wrong way: "You're not thinking of suicide, are you?" That's "leading them to a null answer," says Brian Ahmedani, director of psychiatry research at the Henry Ford Health System. "Saying the question that way says, 'I want you to say no.' And, even further upstream, it tells the patient, 'I don't even want to know about it if you are.' I mean, who's going to say yes, you're having that problem, when someone's led you?"[11]

Yes, suicide is scary. But it's okay: there are guides available that walk clinicians through, word for word, how to ask a patient about it. One is called the Patient Health Questionnaire (PHQ-9) and it's just a check-the-box list of nine questions.[12] (I've gotta say, though, that the suicide-related question is terribly worded: "Over the last two weeks, how often have you been bothered by thoughts that you would be better off dead or of hurting yourself in some way?" At first glance it sounds like you're asking if the person has been bothered by thoughts she'd be better off dead OR be better off hurting herself. And every reporter knows double-barrelled questions are the devil: the interviewee is going to pick whichever's easier to answer—in this case, I'd go for hurting myself as the easier option to cop to. But also, thinking you'd be better off dead is not the same as wanting to kill yourself or thinking about doing it—the latter is much more active and, I'd argue, far more lethal.)

I've heard a lot of clinician variations on the suicide question. "Have you been having thoughts that life is not worth living?" was one of my psychiatrist's favourites, along with, "Have you been thinking of ending your life?" Another psychiatrist favoured "Do you feel safe?" which sounds more like the kind of thing I'd ask myself before heading out on my bike at night, or that I'd ask a Muslim friend living in the United States in 2019. My bias favours compassionate bluntness: Have you been thinking about killing yourself? And, if the answer to that one is negative: Have you wanted to die at all in the past X days/weeks?

Yes, it's uncomfortable to discuss. But the stakes are too high not to.

There are times when wanting your own death is seen not as pathological but as a rational decision, a choice to which you are entitled. It's telling, though, that the kinds of pain North American society acknowledges as so unbearable as to make death an acceptable choice don't include the pain caused by mental illness. In Canada and in some US states, a doctor can legally help you die if you have terminal cancer, but not if a mental illness is wrecking your life. That could change—there will likely be court challenges of the mental illness prohibition on medically assisted death—but a proper discussion of what that might look like, of how a doctor would distinguish between a desire to die driven by a disorder's skewed thinking and a desire to die driven by a rational assessment of what a disorder is doing to your life, is beyond the scope of this book. It is no doubt a question society will have to answer: Why does the pain of people who are crazy carry less weight than the pain of those who are not?

• • •

TREATING DEBILITATING DEPRESSION without addressing suicidality is "like treating a heart attack by saying someone needs to lose weight," Ahmedani says. "If you only treat the weight loss . . . and you don't also put them on cholesterol medication, give them nitro, give them other types of interventions for the heart attack . . . it may not be effective."

If changing the way you do things to drastically improve the answers to such questions as "Will patient kill herself?" and "Will patient cycle in and out of the emergency room dozens of times before killing herself or being indefinitely institutionalized?" isn't your style, there are a few basic changes that could make a difference.

For one thing, stop it with the stupid "no-suicide contracts." Yes, this is a real thing: you make a sick person sign a paper saying they'll stop doing the thing the illness keeps making them do. They're about as effective as telling someone with cancer to stop letting their cells reproduce in a disorganized and uncontrollable way. Some institutions implement these kinds of contracts because it makes them feel better from a liability perspective, as though they're less likely to be sued if patients kill themselves because they made them promise not to kill themselves. Spoiler: this ass-covering gambit does nothing to cover your ass. If someone can prove you knew or should have known a patient was a danger to themselves, you're open to litigation. Especially in the US. It can also destroy any trust between a suicidal person and their clinician if the clinician gives the sense that any such behaviour will be met with punitive action. The prospect of being accused of breaching a contract, legally unbinding as it may be, certainly wouldn't encourage me to open up. "Patients know that it's only a piece of paper and that signing that is not going to change the fact if they're in a desperate place," Tom Ellis says. "It's just so naive on the surface, it's hard to imagine it took hold the way that it did."

If all this sounds like it should be a given, you haven't talked to people who've been the loudest self-harm authorities in popular culture over the past half-century—those who think the mere mention of suicide is enough to send people plunging off cliffs like angsty lemmings. This queasiness is closely connected to contagion theory—the idea that exposure to the very concept of self-inflicted death will cause others to commit suicide when they wouldn't have considered it before. That mentioning or publicizing suicide will lead impressionable individuals—kids and teens, especially—to just off themselves, has been dogma for decades. People refer to the "Werther effect," after Goethe's eighteenth-century novel *The Sorrows of Young Werther* in which the protagonist kills himself—and which, supposedly, gave rise to a slew of copycat suicides across Europe. Even academic researchers have had to confront ethics boards who have freaked out at the thought of talking to suicidal people about their suicidal thoughts for fear that would result in lots of suicides. "This is a common concern," Tom Ellis tells me. "It doesn't happen." He maintains that people actually tend to be relieved to be able to talk about something that is so consuming them. (Yep: I can confirm.) "This is on their mind anyway. It's not something we're creating out of thin air."

The truth is, it's complicated. A 2014 study of dozens of teen suicide clusters (a cluster being anywhere from three to eleven deaths) between 1988 and 1996 found that suicides that received prominent, detailed newspaper coverage—especially celebrity or teen suicides—were more likely to be followed by a "cluster" of three or more teen suicides.[13]

The first thing that came to my mind on reading this study: whoah, teens read newspapers! (And it's killing them in awful ways!) But seriously—even here, causation's tough to suss out: only a quarter of the communities where the suicide clusters occurred had local coverage of that first suicide. That suggests that most clusters happen without prior precipitating coverage.

It's also important to keep in mind, I think, that the suicides in this study took place well before social media and the internet were a thing. It's become easy to find websites and forums where suicide is glorified, where you're given a how-to, without ever having to pick up a newspaper. "It's much harder [for us] to do research with social media. It's so amorphous," Madelyn Gould, an epidemiologist behind the suicide cluster study, tells me over the phone. "There are a lot of causes and the media definitely has an impact but so does just hearing about [suicide], being exposed to it if you're vulnerable."[14]

News coverage still matters but not always in the way you might think. There was a *decrease* in suicides immediately after Kurt Cobain's death.[15] The weeks following a pair of highly publicized teen suicides in the Ottawa region in 2010 and 2011 saw a spike in the number of young people presenting to a children's hospital emergency department for mental health reasons. The seriousness of their conditions hadn't worsened, though, suggesting extensive but sensitive media coverage that emphasized the role mental illness plays in suicide may have spurred kids and their families to seek help, enabling more youths to receive needed services.[16]

Mario Cappelli studied the incident. "You could not have publicized those two deaths any more than they were publicized and we had no increase in suicides. Media . . . talking about suicide keeps mental health at the forefront, right? And that's not a bad thing."[17]

Sensationalistic reporting is always irresponsible; if you can't report on something empathically, compassionately, contextually, you shouldn't be a reporter. Are there irresponsible ways to talk openly about suicide? Of course. Valorizing, glorifying, referring to "successful" suicides versus "failed" ones; talking about someone's bravery in killing themselves—none of that shit helps. Don't do it. It should be common sense not to rhapsodize a tragic death resulting from a debilitating disorder. And, for all the suicide reporting guidelines out there, there are legitimate ongoing concerns about what constitutes responsible coverage. Some news orgs provide contact information for crisis lines and similar at the end of their suicide-related stories, which strikes me as a good and useful idea but it's no substitute for good journalism.

Madelyn Gould believes the key is to approach suicidal ideation as a *treatable symptom* of mental illness rather than a way to solve a problem or the reasonable, inevitable resolution of a shitty situation. "I definitely wouldn't want to see it on the front page. And I wouldn't want to see extensive coverage." Here is where we differ: I believe it's possible to responsibly put suicide on A1 and to portray it, as Gould suggests, as a failure of treatment rather than a glamourized or sensationalized end. (She also thinks stories on the front page should be about hope and recovery. Maybe we need more of that. But bad news is still news; it's our job to make sense of it.)

What galls me is the way contagion freak-outs infantilize human beings with agency. The urge to kill oneself arises from deep-seated despair that goes beyond any blip in public discourse or news cycle obsession. Andrew Solomon in *The Noonday Demon* likens suicide contagion to a hungry person seeing a restaurant and going inside.[18] With all due respect, this makes no sense to me: even if the hungry person doesn't see the restaurant the hunger persists; and if it persists she will probably feel impelled to sate it. Pretending she isn't hungry, acting as though this hunger will go away on its own as long as no one acknowledges its existence, does no one any favours. For no other public health crisis in the world would you suggest that ignoring its toll would make everything better. But for a long time, that's how the media approached suicide.

HOW PREVALENT IS the stone-in-your-gut feeling, the nonplussed sense of loss, of having someone you care about kill themselves? I'll never forget the wonderful woman at Pfizer's switchboard who answered one of my first requests for an interview with the big pharma company, and who sounded as if she was all ready to pass me on to someone who would shoot down said request, but stopped as soon as I told her what I'd be asking about.

"This is a really, really, really important and great topic. I had a friend who killed himself a couple years ago and I'm always trying to figure it out. It touches everybody, so I'm always interested in what kind of insights people can come up with. Because, to me, I'm still left with the idea that he didn't mean to, you know? I mean, he was just overwhelmed, and that's sort of what happened.

"So. I'm going to redirect your call."

26

Certifiable

Picture in your mind a mental hospital, a psychiatric ward, an asylum for the insane. If you grew up in North America in the mid- to late-twentieth century, *One Flew Over the Cuckoo's Nest* probably comes to mind first. Maybe you also think of the film *Girl, Interrupted*. (Remember when Angelina Jolie, as edgy fascinating pseudo-sociopath, was still something of an unknown quantity?) Maybe you read Janet Frame's chillingly good stories, based on her own psychiatric incarceration, of New Zealand madhouses, or *Life* magazine's depiction in "Bedlam 1946" of torturous conditions in American mental hospitals—men and women beaten to death by staff, half-starved, crowded into under-resourced institutions. Maybe you were struck by nineteenth-century woodcuts of people naked, chattering, wild-eyed, chained to the wall and wallowing in their own filth.

The imprinting of those images on the collective psyche drove decades of deinstitutionalization—an en-masse emptying of those long-term facilities for disordered minds. It also drove trans-institutionalization, as legions of people with mental illness were discharged to the street and, without necessary care, were arrested and ended up filling prisons instead.

The idea was to replace that inpatient treatment with outpatient community resources to get people care before they got seriously ill enough to need inpatient treatment. At the time, advances in psychiatric medicine seemed guaranteed, population-level prevention of mental illness a real possibility. It didn't work out that way: in 1960s America, legislation intended to drastically draw down (state-funded) psych hospitals and establish (federally funded) community mental health centres resulted in much more of the former than the latter. Community resources couldn't meet the needs of severely ill people who were now, in many cases, left on their own; where the needed resources existed, the links between hospitals and outpatient facilities did not.[1]

More than half a century later this remains the case. And now the pendulum's swung the other way. It's become fashionable for many clinicians and public health experts to decry society's aversion to housing crazy people in places that'll keep them safe from society and—more to the point—society safe from them. The latter argument has been emphasized by doctors like E. Fuller Torrey, whose book *American Psychosis* laments the lack of institutions, bolstering its argument with a parade of anecdotes and statistics of the grisly crimes committed by violent crazies. (Yes, as discussed, these individuals comprise a minuscule minority of people with mental illness, who are far more likely to be victims of crime than its perpetrators. But don't mess with the narrative.)

Meantime, many jurisdictions, including Canada and the United Kingdom, are coercively treating people at a much greater rate than they did a decade ago, when most of the people filling Ontario's psychiatric hospital beds were there of their own volition. That's no longer true: between 2008 and 2016 involuntary admissions rose 82 percent. Between March and December of 2016, a thousand people a month were hospitalized against their will because of a mental illness.[2] There are different flavours of coercive care and each one is increasing.

Time for some stats. Deep breath: this is important. In Ontario the number of people put on a Form 1 (the seventy-two-hour hold I was put on after my first attempt) jumped 62 percent in eight years.

The number of people put on a Form 3, the two-week forcible stay I was put on, increased 63 percent. Month-long forced stays, Form 4, more than doubled during that time. The number of admissions per patient also rose, which means more people are being hospitalized against their will multiple times a year. Overwhelmingly, they're there because they pose a danger to themselves or are deemed unable to care for themselves—not because they pose a danger to others. The use of involuntary hospitalization is rising most steeply among the young.[3]

You still have rights when hospitalized against your will—you have a right to a lawyer to help you challenge your committal, for one thing. You still have the right to refuse treatment, although that can be formally taken away. And the percentage of psychiatric inpatients being forcibly *treated* has also risen: its share of admissions increased about 15 percent over eight years. But coercion in one domain bleeds into others: part of the reason I agreed to start taking antidepressants despite my—admittedly irrational—misgivings was because I knew my release from hospital, my return to work was contingent in no small part on my good behaviour, on my impressing upon my captors that I was truly trying to get well. I know I'm not the only person who's made that calculated, pressured choice.

These are big increases. And a big deal if the rights to freedom of movement and integrity of the person matter at all.

The trend holds true in British Columbia, where involuntary hospitalization jumped 54 percent in seven years and went from representing the minority to the majority of all psych inpatients. Here, too, they rose most among young girls.[4] It's true in Alberta, Saskatchewan, Manitoba and Nova Scotia. It's true in England, where compulsory hospitalization increased 64 percent in two decades.[5] It's true in Germany, France, Austria and Finland.[6]

As compulsion rises, it discriminates: people involuntarily hospitalized are more likely to be poor, unemployed, less educated;[7] they're more likely to live in poor areas;[8] they're more likely to be persons of colour. Black people in England are almost three times more likely to be involuntarily hospitalized than white.[9] In Ontario, Black people are also over-represented among people placed on Community Treatment Orders, which impose mandatory conditions on your discharge from hospital, requiring you to take your meds, attend appointments and follow doctor's orders or be committed.[10] This disparity could be because people with crappy access to care to begin with are more likely to deteriorate to the point at which coercion becomes necessary. It could be because we more readily rob of autonomy people who are marginalized to begin with. Could be both. It does certainly raise questions about quality of care, equality of care and possible violations of human rights.[11]

What's going on with the increase?

It's not entirely clear. But we can see that in some jurisdictions the number of coerced psychiatric hospitalizations is rising as the number of psychiatric hospital beds drops.[12] The flipped ratio between voluntary and involuntary admissions is fairly intuitive— when you have fewer beds they're going to go to the most acute cases, and those are often going to be the ones that need or are seen to need hospitalization against their will. People may be trying to get into hospital voluntarily only to be turned away. But the absolute number of psych inpatient admissions has gone up, too. People are being hospitalized more often: involuntary visits per patient are up. And more people are deteriorating to the point where they won't seek treatment even if they desperately need it.

In a fee-for-service model of care, there's also a financial incentive: physicians in Ontario get $105 for filling out a Form 1. I'm loath to think doctors are depriving people of their freedom to make a buck, but hospital-level anomalies suggest the question has to be asked.[13]

ANITA SZIGETI'S NAME strikes fear in the hearts of people who commit people for a living. The Toronto lawyer and staunch civil liberties advocate agrees insufficient beds and other treatment resources are at issue but her solution is less compulsion, not more.

Her job is to fight for her clients' rights and autonomy against those who would hospitalize or treat them against their will for their own good. She challenges committals at Ontario's Consent and Capacity Board, seeking to emphasize her clients' civil liberties ahead of the state's responsibility to help people who can't help themselves. She's notorious enough among Toronto-area shrinks that when my psychiatrist saw her name on a book I was reading (*A Guide to Consent and Capacity Law in Ontario* is no beach read, but is very thorough), his eyebrows rose. She is busy. But she is not popular. Where psychiatrists see a necessary, underutilized way to improve the lives and prognoses of people who don't know their lives need improvement, Anita Szigeti sees a set-up stacked against the most vulnerable patients who, no matter how severe their illness, still have rights that are all too easily ignored.

She contends in our chat that most of her clients shouldn't be committed to begin with. Many are held for reasons outside their control and outside the elements of their illness—they don't have housing to go home to, for example, or can't access intensive out-patient treatment that could keep them out of hospital. And anything more than a few days' institutionalization can make you lose the supports you had when you were out, making it even riskier to discharge you: you can lose social assistance, lose your apartment, lose your job, lose touch with whatever social connections you had on the outside. "I don't blame the doctors; they're clinical caregivers. They want their patient-client to get better. They think they can help them."[14]

Psych wards are no longer Bedlam caricatures or Nellie Bly's madhouse. Inpatients have rights and, more importantly, provisions are in place for maintaining them. (Whether those provisions are followed to the letter is another story.) There are protocols for the ways you're treated and what you're treated with and, overwhelmingly, the people who work in those wards—in my limited experience and from what I've heard of others'—are decent and compassionate individuals. But in some ways the places we put the insane still fit Ken Kesey's stereotype. The longer-term ward I stayed in featured putty-coloured floors and walls and ceilings, doors that didn't close and windows that didn't open but were crosshatched with metal mesh nonetheless. There was a common area with tables for eating or playing board games and a smaller alcove with a TV mounted near the ceiling whose channels were the purview of the tall. Windows fitted in the doors to patients' rooms and outside light switches made it easy for nurses to check on you at odd hours of the night, cutting short whatever scrap of sleep you could summon. The mandatory activities were self-parodies, as were weekly meetings where patient-inmates sat in a circle and discussed living conditions. Years later the hospital built a new lounge with money from a generous donor—games, better couches, books, Ping-Pong. Ping-Pong! I cannot adequately express my happiness that this exists.

HOW DO YOU decide when someone's too crazy to make decisions? My most naked personal bias in this regard is decidedly libertarian. I want to throw open auto-locking psych-ward doors and cry, "Go free, crazy people!" But I've spoken with enough disconsolate relatives and health care workers, and seen enough devastating sequelae of treatment foregone, to understand why this is a bad idea.

So how do you make that assessment? Take, as an example, the state of Arkansas, which requires past non-compliance with treatment in order to involuntarily hospitalize someone who poses a danger to himself or others, or whose inability to treat herself and impaired understanding of the need for treatment puts her in danger of deterioration. Colorado adds the possibility that a person "cannot manage resources or conduct social relations," or that they're losing a caregiver. (If having trouble socializing was enough to get a person forcibly hospitalized, I doubt there'd be many people walking free.) Hawaii includes people in danger of inflicting "substantial emotional injury to others." (Um, who isn't?) In New York State, involuntary hospitalization requires a person pose a danger to himself or others, require "essential" treatment AND be unable to fully grasp why.[15]

It's hardly a hospitalize-the-crazies extravaganza, although I know plenty of online commenters who think it should be.

Depriving someone of some rights means you have to be even more vigilant about protecting the rights they still have. But clinicians do sometimes fail in that regard. A March, 2019 report from British Columbia's ombudsperson found the province's hospitals were ignoring the rights of people involuntarily hospitalized. Legally required forms were missing, late or improperly completed. Sometimes physicians failed to explain why the person met the criteria for involuntary admission. Most involuntary patients got no rights advice form, and many had no chance to consent to their treatment.[16]

A slip as simple as failing to fill out paperwork properly can trap you. In my second time through the psych ward post-suicide, the statutory countdown to my freedom should have started on my admittance to hospital. No one filled out that paperwork. The countdown on my Form 1 only started a day later, as I got settled in my curtained-off psych-ward abode. The prospect of another seventy-two hours without natural light or fresh air, after having spent the previous twenty-four hours hospitalized and the forty-eight before that holed up in my apartment ("Yes, but whose fault was that, Anna?" "Not helpful, Mom.") was too much to countenance. Seventy-two hours is an eternity. And no, it isn't the same as spending an entire weekend in your apartment because going outdoors is too much effort: in your apartment you're left to your own devices and you feel like you're there by choice, even if the choice is pathological. And, in your apartment, there's a motherfucking window. In theory I could have appealed my committal to the staff psychiatrist. But it was a Saturday afternoon, and I felt badly about it—I knew enough to know that the psych on call over the weekend is usually swamped.

Late Sunday afternoon I lucked out, as someone persuaded the harried on-call individual to come visit the ward's whiny patient-inmate. I promised not to run away or dash into traffic, to stay as a voluntary patient for as long as my doctor(s) felt necessary, if he would just take me off that Form. He acquiesced. I can't overstate how validating that felt. I was still a crazy person housed in a modern-day loony bin, talking to nurses and social workers about my Thoughts and Feelings and answering daily suicidality questionnaires. But now I could wear pants. I could come and go at will, as long as I informed my keepers where I was headed and when I'd be back, checked in at shift change and didn't abscond for more than a couple of hours at a time. More than that, I regained a sense of agency: I was a competent adult making my own decisions about my health care. If this comes across as semantic nitpicking, you've never had your autonomy snatched or curtailed because you're too nuts to be trusted. Later I asked my psychiatrist why I wasn't offered that same voluntary inpatient status after my first suicide attempt. He said I'd have been a bad candidate for it: I'd made clear I wanted to leave and was at too high a risk of killing myself to be taken off the Form. He then astonished me by saying he probably wouldn't have taken me off the Form the second time around, either, for the same reasons. Yes, I had said I wanted to stay, but I had just made a serious suicide attempt and had a history of similar. It wasn't that he didn't trust me, he said: he didn't trust the mood disorder. The news that my psychiatrist would have kept me locked up came as a blow. It also made me all the more grateful to that doctor who'd made the risky but, for me, enormously life-ameliorating call to set me free.

Apparently you can make psychiatric advance directives—instructions about what to do, where to take you, what your wishes are should you descend into psychic crisis. You can designate power of attorney or a substitute decision-maker who calls the shots when you can't; you can specify treatment preferences. "It's basically the same instrument for health care decision-making that would authorize a living will," says Jeffrey Swanson, who is a psychiatry and behavioural sciences professor at Duke University in Durham, North Carolina. Except you're still alive when people are supposed to follow your directives. "They're basically designed for people who lose capacity to consent to their own treatment and to give people the ability to plan ahead."[17] In the US, about twenty-five states have some kind of legal framework governing psychiatric advance directives. They also have override features.

But take note: if you're rushed to emerg after a serious suicide attempt, no one's going to respect your "Do not resuscitate" directive. I've asked both my own doctor and others about this beguiling option. No dice.

But I figure these directives' limited legal weight is outweighed by the act of writing them. It lets people assert a degree of control over something disturbingly outside their control. "It's the empowering function of sitting down and documenting, ahead of time, your own preferences," Jeffrey Swanson says. "It's kind of like a psychiatric resume—what you look like when you're in a crisis, who should be notified, what medications you're allergic to.... Even if they never used it, they feel more empowered. Just like you might feel better having an insurance policy even if you never use it."

Subsumed by such an agency-stealing disease, we need all the empowering we can get.

THERE ARE A MILLION indignities involved in being hospitalized against your will but one thing that came up in my interviews with both the committed and the committers was that there are *degrees* of crappiness when it comes to losing your freedom in this way. It's unpleasant but it doesn't have to be degrading. It's agency-thieving but shouldn't mean losing your right to due process.

DEANNA

Deanna remembers the darkness of the psychiatric hospital in Kingston, Ontario, where she spent the better part of four years. Not from an absence of windows, although what portals there were, were barred. But a dark greying sense of remove from the outside world.

And a disquieting quiet that her three children pierced when they raced down the long echoing grey hallway that was almost always empty. Mandatory activities included cooking and enforced socialization that she only periodically had the energy for. The ancient elevator creaked each time she took it to the hospital basement for electroconvulsive therapy.[18]

She was paralyzed with fear of being admitted not just to a psychiatric ward, but an entire hospital dedicated to the care and warehousing of the mentally ill. Institutionalization was terrifying on its own but the prospect also reinforced her conception of herself as unwell, unfit, unable to care for those she loved or be the person she thought she was. "I couldn't imagine that that was me and my life— that things had fallen apart to the extent that I needed hospitalization. Not only did I not trust myself, in terms of my safety and my care, but my doctor didn't."

Deanna's first stint as a psychiatric inpatient lasted nine months before she showed a marginal improvement and went home. "But it didn't last. I was only home for about six weeks and then I was back to hospital."

So it went. Deanna figures she lived in hospital for 85 percent of the subsequent four years, exhausting a glossary of drugs and other treatments.

"I couldn't do anything. It was hard to get dressed. It was hard to shower. It was hard to eat." She'd set out on a staff-chaperoned walk outdoors with other patients, along the shore of Lake Ontario, only to find herself depleted within a block and escorted back inside.

LESLIE

Of her first New York City psych ward, Leslie recalls Band-Aid-brown walls, ceiling, floors. No handles or doorknobs. She lost her privacy and her phone and, with it, any lifeline to her loved ones outside the hospital.

"The environments they put you in would make you want to kill yourself, too," she tells me. "There you are, in a room, there's nothing on the wall to look at, it's plain and it's old and the paint's chipping, there's no curtains on the wall 'cause they're afraid you're going to hang yourself. It's convent-style living without a cross on the wall, 'cause they're afraid you're going to jab someone's eye out. . . .

"Imagine, if you can, how demeaning it is to be in this hospital room that is so banged up and then walk into a shower that is covered with mould and there is only cold water, no hot water."[19]

Always, there were roommates. Some better than others: Leslie found herself living beside "a lovely, lovely woman" who thought she was a high-powered insurance firm executive; another said she was a go-go dancer. But the lack of privacy and the prevalence of sleep-filching noise were a nightmare. "There was one woman next door to me that would throw furniture against the wall at night. . . . And there's some that just roam around the hallway babbling to themselves and they don't control them. You can't sleep. You literally can't sleep in those circumstances. They wake you up every half hour. You can't recover."

CINDY

Cindy isn't sure she wanted to die when she slit her wrists in her dorm room in the first semester of college in Iowa but it was enough to get her under round-the-clock scrutiny in a psych department affiliated with her school.

"Oh god, it was terrible. . . . I was under suicide watch, so they had to come check on me every fifteen minutes. I was not allowed to shower alone. There was a phone in my room but the cord was extremely short—I had to sit at the desk hunched over to make any calls. . . . I remember one of the girls that was there, she too had a lot of cuts and scars on her arms. Hers were much worse than mine and I remember sitting there thinking, 'I shouldn't be here.'"[20]

MULTIPLE TIMES EVERY day Andrew Lustig has to decide whether the person in front of him is too unwell and too unable to understand their own unwellness and in too much danger as a result to be let out on their own. The psychiatrist at Toronto's CAMH works in an urban psych emerg with a large number of acutely ill patients. His office is in a building whose halls are blocked off by auto-locking doors and when I visit, the patients I see—mostly men—seem more out of it than dangerous.

"The most important question you answer in the emergency department is, 'Do they stay or do they go?' and that really hinges on the issue of risk: How risky is this person, and what bad things are likely to happen if they leave the hospital today?"[21]

It's a tricky calculation. He wants to get at not just why and how they ended up in the psychiatric emergency department that day, but also at their history of mental illness and of hospitalization. Have they been in treatment? Have they been in hospital before? Have they harmed themselves or others in the past? Like any good journalist, he tries to get multiple sources to create a picture—the person themselves; whoever brought them to hospital if they didn't come on their own; any close family or friends he can track down. He'll ask if the person has been thinking of killing themselves, whether they're planning on doing it, how they'd do it. He'll watch the person closely to see if their affect and behaviour match their words. Invariably they'll have an agenda: either they want to be admitted or they don't, and they'll act and answer questions accordingly. So Lustig listens to what they say but doesn't take their word for it.

Doctors don't have much time to decide whether to put someone on a seventy-two-hour hold, so often that commitment is out of an abundance of caution, he tells me—to keep someone safe in case they may harm themselves, but just as importantly, to give clinicians the chance to observe the person under a great deal of stress. You learn a lot about someone by how they cope in that kind of crisis hospital environment, where they're deprived of their belongings and their ability to smoke or decide when to eat and when to sleep.

It's at this point in the interview that I learn that while CAMH, like my hospital, doesn't let anyone on a seventy-two-hour hold outdoors even on escorted trips, it does let them wear real clothes. You can keep your own clothes?! You can hear, in my audio recording of our conversation, my poorly masked incredulity, my indignation still fresh more than two years after I was denied my own clothing while certifiable. "It's interesting," he muses. "I spoke to an ethicist about that here once and they said they thought that was unethical to take away somebody's clothes. It's quite dehumanizing to have to wear the hospital clothing." YES. Thank you. I brought this up later with my psychiatrist, who said forcing people to wear hospital gowns is a precautionary measure in case they escape: makes them easier to spot.

Many, many, many times, Lustig will let someone go who isn't well, who would benefit from care, but who doesn't meet the legal criteria for committal. It drives family members mad.

"I cannot tell you how many conversations I have with angry families where I'm letting the person go," he says. "The family is yelling at me that they're going to sue me if something bad happens; I just repeat: 'I understand. And I'm sorry. But it's not really up to me—these are the criteria. . . . Just because they're angry or they're going to lose their schooling or lose their house, I'm sorry but I can't detain someone on those grounds.'"

No one likes to admit they make treatment decisions about an individual based on the needs of someone else. But it's inevitable, says Joel Dvoskin, the forensic psychologist. "So if Joe comes in, and is at an acuity level of eight, and I admit him and I settle him down to a five and you say, 'Well, you really should be around a three to get released,' but I don't have any empty beds and at my front door is Sam and he's a ten. . . . There's pressure to release people maybe when you would have rather waited a few days."[22]

"Of course" it's better to get more people into treatment of their own volition, says longtime involuntary treatment advocate E. Fuller

Torrey. But he says the number of people being committed, either on an inpatient or outpatient basis, is reprehensibly low. "I've been told probably two hundred times if I've been told once, 'If you want to help me, doc, just call the CIA and tell them to stop the voice in my head.' . . . So what do you do with someone who has no awareness of their illness?"[23]

Short of death, which is rare but not rare enough, perhaps the most damaging outcome of involuntary hospitalization and treatment is a toxic all-consuming mistrust—of psychiatry, psychiatrists, the medical profession. Of everyone. Of oneself. I'm sure some people emerge from committal in a better mental state and genuinely grateful that someone saved them from themselves, but I know for a fact that coercive treatment sours some people on medicine for life.

Torrey knows hospitalizing and treating someone against their will fosters a lifelong mistrust of psychiatry that means people never seek out or trust a clinician ever again. He contends the benefits of humane coercive treatment for people in need of an intervention outweigh the costs of that deep mistrust, even if he doesn't know how to dispel it.

DOES COERCION WORK?

Depends whom you ask and what you're looking for. Where outcomes are better, it's hard to tell whether you couldn't have gotten that improved result without coercion.[24]

People are less likely to kill themselves while under close supervision in a medical institution than they are outside of it, although hospital suicides do happen: there were 548 deaths in Ontario psych wards between 2008 and 2016, 24 of them suicides.[25] So if you keep someone in hospital when they might otherwise have killed themselves, you've saved a life. And if you frame your choice as being between detention and death, you will err on the side of detention even if the possibility of death is relatively slim. But detention is not without its perils. And there's no control group for a human being: it's impossible to prove someone would have killed herself if set free.

One of the reasons all this is difficult to measure is that a person who doesn't trust their clinicians or lives in fear of getting into trouble with them is unlikely to tell those clinicians when things are going badly. "People do better when they're committed," Joel Dvoskin says, "but it's not clear that they're doing better because of the coercion: it may be that they're doing better because of enhanced services that could have been provided voluntarily."

Then there's the you'll-thank-me-for-this-later trump card. "People who are admitted involuntarily, the vast majority of those individuals at a later point will say, 'Yes, that was an appropriate decision,'" says Richard O'Reilly, a psychiatrist in London, Ontario. "I agree we should try to provide service in the community. But our general hospitals, our local community hospitals, are community resources. And their job is to keep people safe."

Not everyone rages against being forcibly treated. In a 2013 Huffington Post op-ed, a woman named Erin Hawkes compared a patient without insight into her mental illness to a toddler who thinks it would be fun to play with knives. "Though some psychiatrists rely overly on their psychopharmaceutical powers, my brain is in fact too sick to heal on its own," she wrote. "Please, someone, make choices for me when I cannot: choose to give me the treatment that, for me, has worked in the past. Medicate me. Don't leave me to myself; I will play with those knives, and may not learn until I bleed to death what harm I have the 'right' to do."[26]

MENTAL ILLNESS PITS the rights of sick people against the desires of their loved ones more than maybe any other ailment. People want their family members to be taken care of, kept safe; an individual has rights to liberty and, when that is deprived, to integrity of the person unless that, too, is suspended. People want to know everything about what is happening to their loved ones and how they're being helped and what happens next and what else can be done; an individual has rights to privacy, even when that means shutting out the people closest to them. Each jurisdiction has its own rules on when to override a person's privacy, when it's okay to tell confidential things to kin, and who gets to know. I've talked to plenty of family members who've raged against roadblocks to knowing what's going on with the people they love.

Daryl Geisheimer was at his wit's end—he couldn't get a straight answer from the nurses or doctors caring for his son, Brian, in hospital after a suicide attempt, he told a coroner's inquest after his son walked out of hospital and in front of a train. "I was trying desperately to get involved, to volunteer my availability and say, 'I'm surely part of this program. I'm the parent.'"[27]

The system failed Brian and his family at numerous junctures. It appears one of them was communication. But even there, Brian's consent would have been needed to share confidential information with his parents.

It can be a crazy-making trap, trying to get even the most basic information about a loved one who's been spirited into a locked psych ward. It drove my parents nuts, those first few days in hospital and beyond, that sense of enforced helplessness and ignorance: they wanted to be involved in my care—they were there, after all, camped out in hospital for as many hours a day as they were allowed to be— and were told in no uncertain terms that my right to privacy as an adult did not include parental disclosures. "I didn't have any resources," my dad recalls. "We were just winging it. We were desperate. We were frantic. We were scared."

But it's all too easy to override a person's right to privacy when that person is someone unwell whom you love. Mark Lukach's book *My Lovely Wife in the Psych Ward* expresses the enraging heartbreak of caring for someone with severe mental illness better than just about anything else I've read. It also exhibits that easy override: he sits with his wife in the triage room as she answers a nurse's questions on her first emergency department visit, and speaks for her when her answers are unsatisfactory. This is benign and ultimately helpful: his testimony is far more reliable than hers. But it made me squirm: I'd have hated that, were I in her shoes. When she's in remission and he tells her she can't go to a concert because it would involve staying up late and probably driving and, when she resists, retorts, "I do get to tell you what to do,"[28] he is being prudent and probably right but still I winced, vicariously infantilized, yanked back in time to pacing the wet sand on the Lake Ontario beach, yelling at my parents about whether I could be trusted to make decisions.

Here, again, my bias shows. Having something as basic as the right to confidential health information trampled is intensely dis-empowering at a particularly disempowered moment in your life. During my second psych-ward sojourn, my parents met my psychi-atrist. Fine. They came back to visit me in my curtained-off bedspace saying the nice doctor had told them my next treatment option could well be electroconvulsive therapy. I was livid. He'd never mentioned that to me. Even if he had, I wouldn't have been comfortable with him discussing potential treatment pathways with my parents. This probably sounds like an overwrought reaction, and it's largely a matter of principle: I talk to them about all this a fair bit, fairly freely. But on my terms. This small, seemingly meaningless admission was profoundly destabilizing.

SURELY IT'S POSSIBLE for involuntary status to be rendered moot because the patient decides to stay of their own accord. You just need to win them over.

How do you persuade?

Making hospitals less awful would be a start, Andrew Lustig says. Better programming, a comfortable environment, the ability to get fresh air. Some facilities actually have fenced-off green space of some kind where people can go but where they can't run away. (The balcony in my longer-stay psych ward would have made an enormous difference in my quality of life, if only it had been open for more than five minutes a day, or whenever we could prevail on the nurses to let us breathe). Talk to the patient like they're a human being. Like you're on the same side. Try to establish a degree of trust. Explain to them why you want to take whatever interventions you think are necessary, and what you hope that will accomplish. It's not enough to say, "This will make you better." What is better? How will this intervention get you there? In other words, "being empathic—listening, hearing what they have to say, taking an interest in their lives. Not just walking in and saying, 'Here, you need this medication,' but clearly communicating to them you want to help them get better and having them believe that."

Clinical compassion is more crucial here, arguably, than it is in any other field of medicine. Lacking insight into your illness puts you and your doctor at odds from the beginning. "If someone breaks their leg, there's generally agreement between the orthopedic surgeon and the patient that the leg is broken, right? But if somebody has schizophrenia, oftentimes the physician's view is, 'You have schizophrenia.' And the patient's view is, 'I don't have schizophrenia, but people are following me and they want to harm me.'"

That doesn't mean you have to force the patient into things. "The most helpful thing to do," Lustig concludes, "is, I think, to find something where you—the doctor and the patient—can agree on what the problem is. So maybe you can't agree that the diagnosis is schizophrenia, but maybe you can both agree the person is under a lot of stress and that taking this medication will help alleviate the stress."

"DO YOU WANT to spend a few days in hospital?"

It was the first time he'd asked me that. My doctor. In five and a half years of treatment, during which I'd confessed—with 100 percent honesty, I swear—every need for death at my own hand, no matter how fleeting or interminable or nightmare-compelling, whether during insomniac nights or a sudden midday emotional blow to the chest.

We had a deal. One he'd initiated, not me. He'd promised not to commit me. There are few therapeutic gifts more valuable, engendering more trust. Maybe none. It makes it possible, even natural, even therapeutic to tell someone about your desire to kill yourself when you trust them and when they take you seriously and when you know your honesty won't be punished. It made it possible for me not only to tell him I'd stocked up on Aspirin with the intention of overdosing but to pull out the bottle of pills to show him.

So now I was telling him about intense suicidality that commandeered my nights and intruded on my days and my commute and my work, a telescoping anxiety that paralyzed me and convinced me I was in the midst of a psychotic break. (He said I wasn't. So there.) And now he was asking about, offering, an inpatient stay. Because, he said, he figured I wouldn't ask for it myself if I wanted it. Which was true but also maybe overly optimistic on his part: I couldn't imagine a return to the short-stay psych unit with my nurse friends who remembered me better than I remembered them. I couldn't conceptualize that as anything but a surrender to misery or, if I was unspeakably lucky, a chance to will myself into endless catatonia— the next best thing, I figured, to total obliteration. Even when the possibility of surrender seemed a relief, the prospect of re-entering the real world after even a short, even a voluntary stay, took so much out of me I could not imagine mustering the wherewithal to do it.

Transitioning from psych ward to real world as an attempted facsimile of a normal person is, for me, like racing to climb onto a train hurtling at full speed. Many people I've spoken with say they checked themselves into hospital because they didn't trust themselves with themselves. It was such a relief, they said, to give this responsibility to someone else. At the very least it offered respite from that oppressive impossible weight. Maybe a chance to recover. And I get that. And I'm so jealous. A respite I understand. But how do I bounce back? I couldn't. I can't.

So I didn't go. And his offer, his question, both petrified and comforted me. Petrified because it was without precedent and because of that it seemed to indicate an unprecedented fear on his part.

"Oh shit. Did I alarm you?"

"Do I look alarmed?"

But if he were not, why would he have suggested I check myself in before I wreck myself?

Comforted, though, because it was such a respectful way to ask a scary thing. He didn't tell me. He didn't even say he thought I should. He just asked. This, again, was its own invaluable gift.

A doctor's orders needn't come across as orders.

"I think, as a profession, psychiatry has probably lost a lot of its ability to just talk to the clients," Anita Szigeti tells me. "And I think we're definitely seeing force and forced medication where we don't need to, if a doctor had better skills at just therapy and communication."

ABBY'S FIRST-EVER PSYCHIATRIC session ended with her being hospitalized against her will. She then spent a decade cycling through involuntary hospitalization and involuntary outpatient treatment. I call her Abby; she didn't want any part of her real name used for this project. She'd be discharged, often into homeless shelters, arrested after a burst of rage or erratic behaviour, Formed and hospitalized again. She felt scared and disrespected—as though nobody was listening to her or cared to try. Like a nightmare where you talk, yell, and no sound comes out. The swift loss of agency, the forcible treatment, the physical and pharmacological restraints, left lasting psychic scars. Made her vacuum sense of isolation worse. Poisoned any future therapeutic relationship. Talking to me a dozen years later, Abby acknowledged she had issues with mental illness, anger management. She had breakdowns, would "flip out" and kick walls or mirrors, wave a knife, try to slap doctors away or kick her mom off her hospital bed. She finally got out of hospital for good when she signed—coercively, she argues: What choice did she have?—a

Community Treatment Order agreeing to semi-weekly injections that went on for years until finally her doctor said she'd been doing so well he would let her off the treatment order if she agreed to take a low dose of an antipsychotic (olanzapine, the same one I was on a couple of times) voluntarily. She kicks herself in hindsight for not realizing earlier that her relationship with clinicians could have been collaborative rather than coercive.

She wishes someone had made clear this was an option.

Psych wards can save lives. They can provide a safe place to stabilize and, as they did for me, an on-ramp to longer-term outpatient care. Sometimes some people need to be hospitalized even if they don't want to be. But our use of coercion is increasing and it isn't benign; it's the kind of thing whose consequences you'd want to think twice about.

27

Trust Issues

You can have an awful doctor in any sphere and it can fuck with your trust for life. Surgery sucks. Intubation is awful. Chemotherapy is harrowing. But why is mental illness the only sphere of medicine characterized by a deep mistrust of caregivers and caregivers' profession? Cancer foundations are multi-billion-dollar industries yet it's depression—the world's leading cause of years lost to disability, which boasts no ice-bucket-challenge or money-making marathon, which gets fewer public dollars, and whose practitioners make less than the average medical specialist—that's derided as a marketing-driven capitalist fiction.

LANEY

Trapped in a suicidal morass, Laney's son did the supposedly responsible thing. He told his mom to take him to hospital. She did. He checked himself into a psych ward. As the son of a social worker in Virginia he knew what he needed and what he did not. But then everything went wrong, his mom says. The staff was domineering, locked him in seclusion for asking, jokingly, if a grumpy-looking staff member needed a hug. Eventually he unlocked the door with his credit card, walked out and asked to speak with the head nurse—and for a copy of his rights. They tried to grab him; he ran; they took him down, put him in restraints, forcibly injected him with an antipsychotic. He was committed the next day. His parents attended the commitment hearing, begging for him to be let go. No dice.

His mother still can't quite wrap her head around it. "They beat the shit out of someone who was feeling suicidal and wanted to go someplace safe."[1] The committal still haunts her son, she says. He can't own a gun. An IT and computer systems specialist, he was turned down for a federal job (he was working on contract and trying to jump to a full-time gig) because the committal came up on a background search. He hasn't accepted medication since. He hasn't forgiven her. Refused to talk to her for eight years, then relented and let her visit once a year, on Christmas Day. He has a son now, named after her father. Laney (not her real name) has met her grandson twice. "I guess he felt betrayed. And he thought it was my fault." She doesn't know if he's ever tried to kill himself. If he's ever wanted to. "He basically said, 'I'm never going to tell you again if I feel suicidal.'" She asked me to change her name and not to name him for fear of upsetting him.

She hasn't forgiven herself. "Frankly, I don't blame him for feeling like I had led him into the lion's den. As much as it breaks my heart, I don't blame him. I wish I hadn't done it. I wish I had said to him, 'Let's keep you at home and I'll keep you safe at all costs.' It would have kept his dignity. It would have kept his humanity and his self-determination. It would have accepted who he is as a person."

She certainly hasn't forgiven the health structure that did that to him. "And what happened to my son is nothing compared to other people. Nothing." She knows. She started out as a social worker in what she calls a "mental health ghetto"—an area where people were discharged from psychiatric wards into an abyss, sans supports: single-room occupancy units or group homes or the streets. Now her advocacy for the most vulnerable mentally disordered individuals runs counter to a system she sees failing, abusing and infantilizing them in ways that border on criminal.

During a placement for her master's degree in social work, she says, she got an "eye-opening" look at the gap between the advocacy work that interested her and the care-provision that was the status quo: "The 'I know best for you; I know what you need better than you do.' . . . I was confused about how to make it a more empowering experience for such a damaged population."

She became a shit-disturbing crusader, "muckraking with hospitals," pushing for better community care and going after what she saw as systemic screw-ups in the state mental health systems where she'd gotten her start. She briefly headed Virginia's chapter of the advocacy-oriented but largely institution-friendly National Alliance on Mental Illness, but moved on to work at the more radically psychiatry-skeptic National Coalition for Mental Health Recovery.

What Laney preaches is itself not so different from what many public health advocates want to see: more robust community-based outpatient care. "We believe in intervening before it's too late."

But she's sick of seeing mental health budgets swell and ebb like tides pulled by the force of political moons. She's sick of the merry-go-round of one-off funding infusions that never last long enough to change much. She's sick of coercive care, and to her, now, all psychiatric hospitals are inherently coercive. "They just are, under the best of circumstances. . . . I am opposed to inpatient care. I think there's no way to fix it." She's sick of clinician attitudes to people deemed mentally ill. "I despair at the mindset of other mental health professionals—particularly in inpatient settings. And I think that, you know, coercion and 'You will do what I say' and 'I know better than you do' and 'You're behaving badly so I'm going to punish you for it,' I think it's really nearly impossible to get rid of that mindset." For this reason more than the myriad shortcomings and side effects of the best-intended treatments, "survivors don't want anything to do with psychiatric services." She's sick of families supporting laws expanding involuntary hospitalization or treatment because they see no other hope for their loved ones (or themselves). "Families have been so completely failed by the mental health system that they have concluded that forced treatment is the only way to help their family members get better. I don't think family members understand what actually happens" when people are committed. "They have no idea the nightmare has just started for their loved ones." And she's sick of people calling psychic suffering a sickness. Sees it as one more thing pushing coercion: "If you're sick, you can't take care of yourself. You're a helpless person. I don't call them illnesses. I would call them conditions."

I've encountered this argument before. I understand the sentiment but now disagree with the conclusion: calling something an illness forces you to take it seriously, to devote resources to it. An illness can be outside a person's control without that person being out of control—therefore untrustworthy, unfit for autonomy—as a result. But when the illness outside your control is a mental one, the crucial differentiation is often blurred.

Much as you might disagree with Laney's conclusions and her indictment of the entire field, it's tough to argue with her mantra for fixing mental health care. "Make it voluntary. Make it attractive. Make it effective. Make it humane."

IT'S NOT UNUSUAL to find extreme psychiatry-skeptics. The Ontario Institute for Studies in Education (OISE) at the University of Toronto, the biggest post-secondary institution in Canada, now has an antipsychiatry scholarship. "Given the overwhelmingly and disproportionate availability of 'regular' scholarships for studying issues related to psychiatry," the scholarship's website reads, "equity and academic freedom themselves require that antipsychiatry scholars, including exceptional ones, have more equitable access to scholarship support."[2]

I know a lot of serious-minded people who think this is a deeply harmful idea. Bonnie Burstow, the author-activist who endowed that scholarship, is not looking for their approval. She wants to see electroconvulsive therapy criminalized, antidepressants and other psychotropic drugs banned, and psychiatry as a field extinguished. The things we call "mental illnesses" are not illnesses, she says, but "problems living." (I can confirm they are most definitely that.) Antidepressants and electroconvulsive therapy are so damaging, she claims, that "if they told you the truth, no one would take the treatment. What psychiatrists do with depression . . . is not only not meaningful, it should be a crime against humanity. Because it takes healthy people and seriously brain damages them for life."[3]

It's understandable for people who've dedicated their lives to caring for those with depression to be less than tolerant of such maddening misconceptions. But strident smackdowns aren't helping. When Charles Kellner at Mount Sinai in New York dismisses people worried about losing memories to electroconvulsive therapy as being silly at best or Scientology stooges at worst, that doesn't win anyone over.

There are reasons why mental illness is a sphere of medicine so characterized by mistrust.

Antidepressants, for example, have a bad rap in large part because clinician, researcher, marketer pronouncements about the way they worked overstated their certainty, simplicity and efficacy.

"I think sometimes, to explain things to people, we have maybe oversimplified things . . . using 'chemical imbalance' to explain things to people, using the analogy of not having enough insulin, etcetera," Husseini Manji, Janssen Pharma's global head of Neuroscience Therapeutic Area and the man behind Janssen's ketamine experiments, admits to me. "I think some of the oversimplification was done with good intent. And I'm guilty of it. Because with things like depression, often people seem to think, 'If I only tried harder. What's wrong with me?' And you almost want to say, 'No! It's not you.'"[4]

No one's known much about depression treatment in the history of treating depression. So once researchers and clinicians found something that appeared to effectively treat depression, they explained it and sold it to governments and the public (and perhaps to themselves) on a reverse-engineered mechanistic explanation that made sense at the time but hasn't held up to scrutiny.

This overstatement of psychiatric certainty when it comes to understanding the way depression works has become one of anti-psychiatry's most effective weapons. Gary Greenberg, author of *Manufacturing Depression* and coiner of the delicious Blakeian phrase "what's dark and Satanic about the depression mills,"[5] isn't afraid to wield it. But when you press him he's cool with the idea of depression as an illness, as long as you don't insist on bringing biology into it. "I actually think an illness, a disease, is better understood as a rhetorical device than as a biological category. It provides us with a way to decide how to allocate social resources: a disease is a kind of suffering that deserves social resources, and social resources can include research, drugs, compassion, money. Is depression a legitimate disease by that definition? Absolutely."[6]

Most psychiatric researchers and clinicians—certainly everyone who specializes in the neurology and neurochemistry of depression—would understandably refuse to abandon the idea of depression as a medical disease with an identifiable (even if as-yet unidentified) pathophysiology, especially as neuroplasticity and neurocircuitry appear to offer potentially illuminating avenues of inquiry. But at the patient level, does it matter? Does it do anyone any good to argue with a patient over the pathogenesis of their illness if your common goal of remission doesn't require anywhere near that unanimity? I talk to my doctor and follow his advice because I trust him, not because he has or claims to have all the answers as to where depression comes from or how it works or even how these drugs work. Arguably he's a better psychiatrist because he's so straight up about his profession's uncertainty.

Paul Kurdyak at CAMH is on board. "A lot of practitioners will say to patients, 'We're giving you Prozac or Zoloft or whatever because it increases the serotonin in your brain and that's what's going to make you feel better.' I think that's a highly reductionist explanation. I say, 'It seems as though you're depressed. I'm going to prescribe a medication that, according to the evidence, has the best balance of efficacy and side effects.' . . . I like saying that, because it's honest."[7]

Gary Greenberg is cool with the idea of psychiatrists psychiatristing, so long as they're forthcoming about what they know and what they don't know and their rationale for pursuing the treatment modalities that they do. "If every psychiatrist would just go and say, 'Okay, here's what your symptoms are: you're not sleeping, you're not eating, blah, blah. The thing that I've found, in my experience, helps those symptoms is this drug. And I have no idea why.' . . . If a doctor was just to do that with a patient, it might diminish the placebo effect but . . . it might also increase trust and intimacy with the doctor and that might actually make their depression better. There might be more honesty. If there's honesty going in one direction there might be honesty going both ways. Who knows?"

But why is it radical—why does it even need stating—that a professional who deals with the most intimate and vulnerable aspects of human selfhood should be honest and open about what they're doing and why? Should treat patients as people, as partners in care, rather than as a flawed mental vessel needing their unadulterated expertise, no questions brooked?

One thing I've heard (and seen) over and over is how much deeper an understanding people have of mental illness once they've gone through it themselves (directly or indirectly via someone they love). Any experience cuts closer when you know it firsthand. It follows that health practitioners care better for depressed and suicidal people if they've been there. But imagine if the only competent oncologists were ones in remission for cancer; if the only decent obstetricians were ones who'd given birth; if only the superannuated could be geriatricians and a neurosurgery prerequisite was having had someone slice into their own brain. Surely the very starting point for trained clinicians in a "caring profession" is basic human empathy—and learning! And putting learning into practice!—to be able to provide adequate, evidence-based mental health care and not be insensitive assholes about it.

Even Bonnie Burstow, who endowed the antipsychiatry scholarship at OISE, agrees that paralytic despair, impenetrable suicidality, psychosis benefit from intervention—she just favours psychotherapy, exercise, social supports over drugs and other medical interventions. The mode of therapy she extols—enlisting suicidal people as "co-investigators" examining their despair and alternate ways out of it—is strikingly similar to that advocated by David Jobes and others pioneering the Collaborative Assessment and Management of Suicidality model. I suggest to her that she's perhaps not so philosophically different from the psychiatrists she holds in contempt. They both recognize something is wrong. They both think things can be done to alleviate the wrongness, to help make life better or bearable. Both favour an intervention, backed by evidence, that puts the patient in the therapeutic driver's seat.

Mistake. "It is a huge philosophical difference to believe things are diseases of the brain and to believe that people have problems living that they need help with. It is an unbelievably big philosophical difference." She pauses. "You haven't read my book, have you?" You know you're in huge trouble, as an interviewer, when someone is asking whether you've read their book. (And, full disclosure, I had not. I've since read several, those she's written and a couple she's edited.)

I do understand the rejection of the very idea of mental illness, a repudiation of any medicalizing of the mind. Many people reject the idea that the things that make them unique creatures are reducible to a series of electric impulses. (Although it sounds pretty gorgeous and cool to me.) And, as a patient, whether you classify the thing ripping you apart as an illness or you don't doesn't change what it does to you and your life; it doesn't change which interventions alleviate the awfulness and which don't. It does, however, change your ability to access interventions and it changes incentives for funding research into new ones. It changes the rules around who provides which interventions and who gets to decide what to call the thing ripping you apart. That's worth making a fuss over.

Illnesses get coverage. Treatments for illnesses get research resources. People with illnesses have a shot at time off work. People with chronic illnesses and disabilities have rights under human rights codes. Philosophical debates and professional turf wars are well and good until they impinge on individuals' ability to get care that works, to get respect and compassion.

Whether or not you believe that chronic mood disorders are the result of a faulty brain, the need to classify these despair-states as illnesses and treat them as such remains.

But people don't seek treatment they don't trust. The most strident, consistent, compelling objections to psychiatry in general and depression in particular—the science is perceived to be a sham; the treatment is seen as harmful and coercive—are rooted in legitimacy. Industry and clinicians have overstated depression drugs' efficacy and oversimplified the way depression works. There are side effects to all medical interventions, some more serious than others. People with mental illness or people believed to have mental illness are hospitalized and treated involuntarily. But none of this means that depression isn't a real, debilitating illness. Depression is a genuine and genuinely awful condition; we just don't understand it. Drugs, psychotherapy, electroconvulsive therapy, repetitive transcranial magnetic stimulation, exercise, all work on some people to some degree. Depression's treatment toolbox remains inadequate. Coercing people into getting care is crappy no matter how necessary it is (and people will always disagree as to what justifies that suspension of basic liberty; this is why recourse is important). What this means is that failing to address psychiatry's credibility problem means people will go untreated or under-treated or die.

"It wouldn't be psychiatry" if it didn't involve losing people's trust, Bonnie Burstow says. I'd like to believe that's wrong. Because if losing trust is a necessary part of a given field of medicine, it is a bad field of medicine.

PATRICK

Patrick had been a mess for more than half his life. On good days, he sleepwalked through the motions; on bad days, he was paralyzed by anxiety and self-recrimination.[8]

It started in Grade 9. He became lethargic, lost energy. Fixated on a growing list of his own shortcomings, things he needed to fix within himself to make everything better. Learned to cope with a subsuming sense of worthlessness by retreating into mental haze. "I was kind of out to lunch," he says. "Normal situations gave me anxiety. So I avoided them."

That fog makes it hard, even now, for him to recall specific events in his past. It's like he's straining to observe the details of someone else's dream. Chronic mental illnesses mess with both the way you perceive your world and your ability to recall it later. Many of my more intrusive personal interviews for this book were exercises in frustration as I prodded people to recall episodes distorted by cognitive biases and glitchy memory systems.

"All I have to do," Patrick told himself over the course of decades, "is solve this endless list of things and then everything will be better. You very much tend to blame yourself for all these symptoms. You feel you're worthless. Yeah, it kind of sucked. But it was just my daily life. I still managed to do things, but I didn't do very well. I didn't really talk to anyone, didn't do well socially, didn't date. Just trying to get through the day. It was a slog, basically. It was a huge slog."

Outwardly, he was coping. Excelling, even. Graduated from university with a degree in political science. Spent years teaching English in Korea, backpacking across Southeast Asia. "I was trying to get away from my problems but I just brought my problems with me. Kind of like wherever you go, there you are."

He worked as a temp for the Ontario government, as a bike messenger, managing an inventory yard at a construction site. Sought treatment when his motivation was robust enough not to be eclipsed by the hurdles and wait lists. Saw a family doctor "who was totally afraid to write any kind of prescription at all," waited five months to see a psychiatrist for what felt like a "weird, useless kind of consultation."

"A lot of psychiatrists are just jerks. Like, they're very condescending. . . . The bedside manner was usually very cold and dry. A lot of them, I couldn't even get a word in. It was a very mechanical kind of process. And those are the kind of people who are telling me to go on medication." How could he trust them?

Patrick went on and off antidepressants for a few years. Mostly off. In part because they never kicked in before his own self-loathing convinced him the issue was himself and his failings—"just a few problems I need to figure out"—not his illness. In part because of a deep-rooted aversion to psychopharmaceuticals reinforced by the information he sought out online.

"You're still afraid of the side effects, even though the side effects really are nothing compared to depression itself. Like, I was talking to one guy on the internet, on a forum. He was in his late thirties, pretty severe depression. I was trying to convince him to try medication, and he was like, 'Yeah, but won't that affect my libido?' Uh, you already said your libido is nonexistent." There's a tendency to think, "'I don't want to be a slave to medication.' People kind of self-sabotage sometimes."

For all his reluctance to put his trust in conventional antidepressants, Patrick's need for amelioration led him to Peru for an ayahuasca retreat.

The plant-derived psychedelic drug has become trendy among the wealthy in search of a wellness fix. In elaborate ceremonies, shamans combine leaves from *Psychotria viridis* with vines from *Banisteriopsis caapi*—mixing serotonin-targeting hallucinogen N,N-dimethyltryptamine with harmala alkaloids that act as monoamine oxidase inhibitors.[9] The same kind of thing, in other words, that I spent years trying, but with an organic substance of uncertain potency and purity consumed in an uncontrolled environment without close medical supervision.

"I started reading on the internet about it. . . . It was all success stories. I was like, 'Wow. This is the real deal.'"

So he went for it. Booked a retreat at a place in the mountains that got rave reviews online. Sat with fellow acolytes in a circle in a yurt, on a mat with a vomit bucket beside him. Drank the psychedelic brew. Results were not as advertised.

"It was a disaster. A complete disaster," he says. "The first time was pretty bad but the second time was a nightmare. I don't even know where to start." He recalls gory imagery, the horrifying feeling he was about to strangle someone to death. He thought, "I'm going to be in a Peruvian mental asylum for the rest of my life." For the first time in all his years of melancholic fog, Patrick says, he felt suicidal. Even back in Canada, he was in rough shape. "Not so much flash-backs as just not being able to handle having really horrible thoughts, not being able to handle life, seeing it as kind of meaningless."

His online search for solutions then led him to ketamine. The party drug was making a name for itself as a potential panacea for treatment-resistant depression. Patrick went to New York to a clinic where an anaesthesiologist administered ketamine intravenously off-label, for a fee.

This cross-border, self-funded test of a relatively unproven treatment turned out better than the last: before the hour-long intravenous drip was even complete, Patrick sat and watched the liquid disappear into his arm and felt . . . better. "My thinking got really rational all of a sudden. Problems that had seemed totally insurmountable suddenly became so easy to overcome."

He felt, briefly, like the conductor of his own brain.

"I didn't hallucinate or anything, but I had this kind of idea that I was in my head and everything was spinning like crazy and I was like, 'Augh, it's really crazy here. Just calm down.' And the spinning got slower and slower and then it was stable. Calm and optimistic. Secure. Social interaction suddenly was very, very easy. Whereas previously it had been incredibly difficult. I could walk into a coffee shop and talk to a barista."

Patrick got three $400 injections over the course of a week before heading back home to Toronto. "I started dating a lot. It's always been something I avoided. You feel like you're the worst person: Why would anyone want to date me? But I was dating up a storm. It was really great." But the awesomeness wore off gradually; within two months, "I felt like crap again, basically."

He tried to find a Toronto doctor who'd give him ketamine and restore that magic feeling. Easier said than done. "People are pretty conservative here. Especially with mental health, people have a hard time. You don't have a bone sticking out of your leg," so there's less a sense of try-anything urgency. Most places he asked, he didn't get past the receptionist. "I mostly just got laughed at. Like, are you crazy? Prescribe ketamine?"

Eventually, he was referred to a Toronto doctor who'd been running trials on ketamine but had since switched to repetitive transcranial magnetic stimulation (rTMS). He joined the trial; it didn't work. He recalls a mechanical arm and a large disc against his head, and a painful sensation "like someone had a fishhook through your head."

But he didn't give up. He got a new doctor. Hearing him describe this individual after his litany of less-than-stellar treatment felt like watching two figures run in slow motion toward each other through a field of wildflowers.

"She was awesome.... She was just super-compassionate. A good listener."

To be clear, this was also the first Canadian doctor who agreed to prescribe him ketamine; people tend to like clinicians who give them what they want. But it still floors me that this dude, after eighteen years of severe depression and a deep distrust of the medical field, waxes lyrical over the prospect of an empathic physician. What a concept!

Now Patrick was getting intranasal ketamine—syringe-type vials with misters attached that he'd spray up his nose once every two or three days. He'd pick up a month or two or three from the one pharmacist in the city that dispensed take-home ketamine (this is not, incidentally, something even the boldest ketamine-boosters I spoke with would recommend you try). "The weirdest part was being high on ketamine every three nights," Patrick says. "It was kind of fun. Especially at first. Just to be able to legally do that is pretty nice."

But the antidepressant effect wasn't there. He got high but remained hopeless. And he was developing worrying signs of dependence—feeling like he needed more, getting antsy as time ticked toward his next dose even as he felt it was now making him physically ill.

Even then he was resistant to traditional antidepressants. "She kept suggesting I try medication again, and I was really stubborn about it." He avoided them for the same reasons he'd avoided them for years—fear of becoming dependent, of being changed in some fundamental way. "I'd just heard about bad reactions. I was very worried about anything that would change my brain chemistry."

Yes, someone who tried to treat his depression with ayahuasca and ketamine, who experimented with LSD in his early twenties, was so fearful of antidepressants' effects on his brain chemistry that he kept refusing to try them even at the urging of the first doctor he'd ever truly trusted. This is not unusual: this is what society thinks of psychiatry and pharmacotherapy. I know plenty of people who'd sooner take mind-altering recreational drugs than anything that operates on those same pathways but comes from a prescription pad and a pharmacy. This trust crisis kills people. Or it destroys their lives when they don't get effective treatment.

"So it took a lot of convincing. [My doctor] just kept bringing it up. She's really great . . . the best person. She just kept subtly implying, maybe it's time to give this up. Maybe we should try something else. At some point I was like, yeah, this isn't working. I'm just getting high."

So he started on escitalopram, the run-of-the-mill selective serotonin reuptake inhibitor I'd tried following my first suicide attempt. "And that actually started to work. Gradually, very slowly, as months went by. . . . And I gradually started to kind of turn my life around." He went back to school. Studied web design. Got a job he genuinely enjoyed. Started meditating on the subway. "It's relaxing, and it kind of organizes your thoughts more. . . . It's like creating your own safe zone in your head. A little bit of distance from what's going on."

Dating is still tough. Self-esteem is still an issue. But "relatively speaking, I'm doing great compared to where I was before."

I'm not the hopey-changey type. But hearing this inspires both a vicarious, celebratory joy and a murderous envy.

I'll have what he's having.

PART V

A DENOUEMENT
OF SORTS

28

First Person Afterword

The worst moment of this chasing was with a woman I met for an interview at a Tim Hortons in Toronto. I arrived late, asked what I could get her. She had the world's most convoluted request: a small black coffee filled all the way up, with an extra cup, and two milks, and a cup of ice water, and a toasted multigrain bun with light cream cheese on the side and cucumber on the side. So I did. But I also, idiot, offered to get her something more—a proper sandwich—so she asked for Tuscan chicken on a bun but they only had chipotle chicken in a wrap so I got the wrap and an extra bun and sat and watched her meticulously deconstruct and reconstruct the food and drink in front of her as I tried and failed to ask her questions. She didn't want to talk. Got upset when I asked anything personal or painful, which was every single question: if she was hoping for small talk and a coffee, she was sitting across from the wrong girl. "Let's just eat first, okay?" she suggested.

A woman who was a patient advocate-liaison affiliated with the Centre for Addiction and Mental Health had put me in touch with her as someone who could talk to me about falling through the chasms in the health system. As she reconstructed her wrap, she asked me about myself, my job, my reasons for writing this book. The first time she asked I said something about the gap in depression discourse, the need for a clear-eyed, critical but measured examination of what we know and don't know and the ways we fail to use the already inadequate resources we have to treat people who need help now, not when we come up with something better. But the second time she asked I mentioned my own experience and she fixated on the first suicide attempt and my time in the psych ward. "But *why* did you try to kill yourself? What was going on in your life? What happened in your childhood?" She decided I must be bipolar, because "I can see you're manic. You're all hyped up. And I know these things. You laugh, but I know." She decided writing this book was a terrible idea—"You aren't well. And asking questions like this, you're going to trigger other people"—and that, moreover, I should march myself into hospital right away because I needed to be committed, maybe for a while. She was in rough shape, struggling with more than just her mind: she was painfully thin—crepe skin stretched over spindly bones as she picked at her food. She'd spent years in and out of inpatient anorexia treatment, being force-fed daily. She said she now had an obstructed colon that prevented her from eating. But her ability to demolish me was masterful. She expertly pinpointed every agonizing weakness in my self-view, every self-doubt that kept me awake at night and paralyzed me in the morning, and prodded each one of them to the point of incapacitation. Finally, an hour and an eternity after I'd sat down, it was almost over. She asked me to walk her to her appointment and then help her find her psychiatrist's office. I stumbled away drunk on self-loathing. I felt crazy and stupid and liable to harm others, driving them, through my clumsy insensitive privacy invasions, to kill themselves. And that's the greatest fear, right? That disclosure will turn against you. That my literary exercise could be responsible, even indirectly, for the anguish or, god forbid, suicide deaths of other human beings.

I needed to talk to Andrew Solomon about how he does it. And why he decided to tell everyone about all this awful personal stuff in his world-shifting book *The Noonday Demon*. He was kind enough not only to respond but also to invite me over for a chat at his beautiful house in lower Manhattan. I brought fresh croissants because I know you can't show up at someone's house empty-handed but then was so agog at his study I left them in their buttery paper bag by my plush chair while we talked and I tried not to ogle the wall-to-wall books too obviously or enviously. He spoke slowly, thoughtfully, as though taking a topic he knew backwards and looking at it anew.

"I think there's a kind of social responsibility to being open and public insofar as you are able to be, and different people are able to be to different degrees. I live in a city, occupy a context and work in a field where I wasn't going to lose a lot of credit because I had been depressed. So I felt like I had less to lose than other people would. If I weren't going to talk about it, then who would?"[1]

He'd also already emerged from one closet and wasn't prepared to spend his life sequestered in another. "I felt that, as a gay person, I had lived a life for quite a while in which I had a secret, and some people knew and other people didn't know, and I'd finally come out of the closet. . . . I had decided I wanted never to have a secret again where I had to wonder, 'Do those people know that those people have told those people?' And I think that, a lot of the time, people who are depressed devote so much energy to secrecy that could be better devoted to getting better."

Truth. The relief I feel from being able to tell people—or even from not having to hide how I'm doing or make up alternative reasons for psychiatric appointments or drugs or impossible mornings—draws me almost as powerfully as the self-destructive fear that disclosure will mean recrimination, will shaft opportunity or connection or prompt polite insidious shunning at best. It's painful. I live in fear I'll regret it. But, often, it's too important not to.

"Telling the whole world can be a stressful operation, and I'm not necessarily recommending it for everyone," he says. "It seems to have worked out reasonably well for me to do so." The response he got has been overwhelming. He figures he gets twenty, thirty emails a week from people who've read his book and want to talk to him about their depression, about their child's or spouse's or sibling's. Seeking help or commiseration: Does he know a good psychiatrist in their small hometown? Can he tell them what drugs might work? Sharing their own stories. "I give them advice within the limits of my ability to give advice....I don't want anyone who feels abandoned by and disconnected from the world to get another experience of abandonment from me. So even when they're people who don't particularly stir my sympathies, I always try to deal with them as kindly as I can and to say as much as I can about helping them."

He tells me that today his bottom-feeder psycho-emotional lows aren't as severe as they once were. His husband and two young kids and their Manhattan house help act as ballast for a forward-moving existence. "I have a much more solid life than I did when [the depressive demons] first came. But, yes. It rears up. And every time it does, it's shocking all over again. I mean, I wrote a whole book about this. I have to give public lectures about it. And I'm still overwhelmed by how painful it is when it comes back again."

It's been almost eight years since I first tried to kill myself and more than four years since I first started poking at the idea of writing a book about this basket-case condition, and there are days I wake up and any possibility of improvement, any chance that I could ever get better, is drowned in the undertow of despair. But not every day is like that. Most days I make it into the newsroom at Reuters, where I work. Most days I work, and it feels good—like I'm building ground beneath my feet even as I struggle to keep from plummeting. I couldn't tell you if I'm any better off than I was the September of my first suicide attempt. I know I've gone through periods, some quite recent, where I was worse. But work on this project gave me something to cling to and build on. It was validating. Almost every interview I did reinforced that this shit sandwich of an illness is genuine and genuinely awful and affects many, many more people than me. Those were days that made it seem worth plugging away.

...

ONE OF THE DANGERS of recognizing that your depression and its dreary behavioural accoutrements constitute an extrinsic pathology rather than intrinsic failure is that, in trying to disentangle what's actually you from what's your soul-destroying disorder, it's tempting to tell yourself that everything you dislike about yourself is due to depression. It's tempting to tell myself I'll get completely better and will be fantastic and personable and accomplished and attractive. And I know that's not how it works. Even if treatment can alleviate the psychomotor retardation that keeps me bedridden, apartment-ridden and slow, I'm not going to magically run marathons. Even if it no longer required wrenching fortitude just to get out of bed and out the door in the morning, I know I'd still have to set multiple alarms and reminders for myself if I'm ever going to be on time. Even if I can someday countenance group social interactions without dread filling my chest like thick cold smoke, I'm not going to be the bubbly life of the party. I'll probably never get rid of self-loathing and self-doubt; but I can try to neutralize their effects.

Brain-stimulating, mind-mapping Helen Mayberg of Mount Sinai's Center for Advanced Circuit Therapeutics sees that. "There are people who think a stimulator [implanted in their brain] is going to give them a life transplant. It doesn't. It takes away depression. So what is it that you imagine of yourself if you weren't depressed? Some people have realistic expectations of what that means. If you haven't worked in five years, you're not going to be CEO of the company that you used to work in the mailroom for. So who do you think you are as you emerge from depression?"[2]

That question can horrify. There are days when I can't conceptualize a self I would want to remain alive to be. Other days I can imagine that person but can't bear the trek it would take to become her. Other days, the trek seems doable.

THIS IS NOT a triumphant book. No one finds herself; no one is saved, although some remarkable people do incredible things. There is no happy ending. It's an uncomfortably personal exploration of a sickeningly common illness no one likes talking about, one that remains under-treated and poorly treated and grossly inequitably treated in part because of our own squeamishness in confronting it or our own denial of its existence as an illness and the destruction it wreaks when left to its own devices.

It doesn't have to be this way. There are pathways to compassion-ate, equitable, informed care for an illness that pummels too many for too long without respite. But we need to act like this is something we care about.

Again and again and again and again, when an interview went from need for reform to methods of reform and then to the public pressure and political will needed to achieve reform, I asked how to muster the latter, and clinicians and researchers threw it back at me: "That's your job."

I'm torn on that front. I'm a journalist, not an advocate or an activist. But I can inform, I can document, I can explore, I can pro-voke, I can punch in the face with words. The topic of depression in the context of my writing this book is complicated by my conflict of interest: I want this stuff to change; I want to change discourse and attitudes and, as a result, alter outcomes. I want someone to come up with new medical interventions that work magic. This dis-order that I have corrodes the sense of self and destroys the desire to live; hope in recovery, of getting "better," diminishes to nothing, a sliver of sandcastle in a rising tide. But if I kill myself, if I don't achieve and maintain remission, it won't be because the system that fails millions daily has failed me: the system's treated me just fine; it just isn't good enough yet.

Our failure to address this illness is a systemic fuckup with an enormous impact; it compounds marginalizations of race and income, and harms most those least able to advocate for themselves. It's inadequately explored and conversation on the subject, as with so many systemic fuckups, is too often dominated by platitudes and siloed extremes.

For a society that's gone so far in so many civil and scientific arenas, there are some things we still do astonishingly badly. Treating the most debilitating chronic illness out there is one of them.

So let's fix this, goddammit, and move on to bitching about something else.

Resources and Further Reading

For immediate help:

> www.crisisservicescanada.ca
> 1-833-456-4566 (in Quebec: 1-866-277-3553)
> or text 45645 between 4 p.m. and 12 a.m. ET

For youth:

> kidshelpphone.ca
> 1-800-668-6868
> Or text CONNECT to 686868
> Or text (778) 783-0177 between 6 p.m. and 12 a.m. PT

For suicide survivor support:

> www.suicideprevention.ca/Survivor-Support-Centres

To learn more about suicide, mental illness and mental health care options:

> www.camh.ca (Centre for Addiction and Mental Health)
> cmha.ca (Canadian Mental Health Association)
> mdsc.ca (Mood Disorders Society of Canada)
> www.nimh.nih.gov (The National Institute of Mental Health)
>
> mindyourmind.ca
> www.suicideinfo.ca
> teenmentalhealth.org

Help Lines:

First Nations and Inuit Hope for Wellness Help Line (24/7)
> 1-855-242-3310

Trans Lifeline 1-877-330-6366

Alberta Crisis Line 1-403-266-4357

British Columbia Crisis Line 1-800-SUICIDE
BC211 Referral Hotline (24/7) Dial 211
Manitoba Crisis Line 1-877-435-7170
New Brunswick Crisis Line 1-800-667-5005
Newfoundland and Labrador Line 1-888-737-4668
NWT Help Line (24/7) 1-800-661-0844
Nova Scotia Crisis Line 1-888-429-8167
Nunavut Line (7 p.m.–11 p.m., EST) 1-800-265-3333
Ontario Crisis Line 1-866-531-2600
Good2Talk Ontario Post-Secondary Student Helpline 1-866-925-5454
Prince Edward Island Crisis Line 1-800-218-2885
Quebec National Crisis Line 1-866-277-3553
Saskatchewan Crisis Line 1-306-525-5333
Yukon Crisis Line (7 p.m.–12 a.m., PST) 1-844-533-3030

Further Reading:

Willow Weep for Me: A Black Woman's Journey through Depression by Meri Nana-Ama Danquah

Freshwater by Akwaeke Emezi

Faces in the Water by Janet Frame

To the River: Losing My Brother by Don Gillmor

American Melancholy: Constructions of Depression in the Twentieth Century by Laura D. Hirshbein

One Flew Over the Cuckoo's Nest by Ken Kesey

My Lovely Wife in the Psych Ward by Mark Lukach

Committed: The Battle Over Involuntary Psychiatric Care by Dinah Miller and Annette Hanson

The Bell Jar by Sylvia Plath

Madness in Civilization: A Cultural History of Insanity by Andrew Scull

The Noonday Demon: An Atlas of Depression by Andrew Solomon

Darkness Visible: A Memoir of Madness by William Styron

All My Puny Sorrows by Miriam Toews

American Psychosis: How the Federal Government Destroyed the Mental Illness Treatment System by E. Fuller Torrey

Prozac Nation: Young and Depressed in America by Elizabeth Wurtzel

Acknowledgements

A reporter's only as good as her sources and here I've been exceptionally fortunate. I want to thank, sincerely and obstreperously, everyone who gave me their time, experience and expertise in my pursuit of this book—everyone who talked to me, met with me, sent me papers, showed me their brain banks, recalled for me the worst moments of their lives. Thank you. You give me reasons to wake up in the morning.

I want to thank my expert readers, geniuses in their fields who took the time to read, comment and give feedback on my manuscript. Irfan Dhalla, Marcia Valenstein, Paul Kurdyak, Sarah Lisanby and Kwame McKenzie—you made this book so much better.

I owe an incalculable debt of gratitude to Louise Dennys, the brilliant powerhouse who brought this beast into being.

To Rick Meier, a stalwart and one of the first to wrestle with this creature, and Angelika Glover, a pro who gets it.

To the arts councils of Toronto, Ontario and Canada, who taught me humility by turning me down for every grant I applied for but one, and to Denis De Klerck, who convinced Ontario to give me $1,500. You were among the first to believe in this thing.

To José Silveira, who teaches me to make life worth living and who, let's face it, puts up with a lot.

To Omar El Akkad, the human being I want to be.

To Brendan Kennedy, who keeps saving my life.

To Richard Warnica, who makes me keep chasing.

To Allison Martell, who inspires me.

To Leslie Young, who keeps me grounded.

To Amran Abocar, who makes a day job possible.

To Jennifer Griffiths, a visual wizard.

And to Heather Cromarty, a true ally.

To Gram, who was right all along, who made me a writer. And to Grandma Ruthie, who shows me what strength is.

To my beloved baby siblings, Daniel and Juliet Paperny, my muses and partners in crime. And to their partners, Lindsay Paperny and Jaylen Gadhia, masters of fortitude. And to Zoe, my little rock star.

And, above all, to my parents, Audrey Mehler and David Paperny, who support me when I need it most and want it least, who teach me resilience through unconditional love and inappropriate jokes.

Thank you.

Notes

CHAPTER 1: CATACLYSM

1. Jayme Poisson and Curtis Rush, "Toronto Police Shoot and Kill Man with Scissors Wearing Hospital Gown," *Toronto Star*, February 3, 2012.

2. Tim Alamenciak and Hamida Ghafour, "Who Was Sammy Yatim?" *Toronto Star*, August 24, 2013.

3. Richard Warnica, "The Life and Bloody Death of Andrew Loku," *National Post*, July 17, 2015.

4. Anna Mehler Paperny, "Ontario NDP Unveils Platform, Includes Corporate Tax Hikes and Contingency Cushion," *The Globe and Mail*, September 25, 2011.

CHAPTER 2: WHEN YOU TRY TO DIE AND DON'T

1. Ontario Mental Health Act, 1990, www.ontario.ca/laws/statute/90m07.

2. www.sse.gov.on.ca/mohltc/ppao/en/Pages/InfoGuides/2016_Form1.aspx.

3. https://www.sse.gov.on.ca/mohltc/ppao/en/Pages/InfoGuides/2016_ Involuntary_Patients.aspx.

4. Heather Stuart, "Violence and Mental Illness: An Overview," *World Psychiatry*, June 2003.

5. Omar El Akkad, "Steve Jobs: The Man Who Changed Your World," *The Globe and Mail*, October 5, 2011.

6. James A. Kruse, "Methanol and Ethylene Glycol Intoxication," *Critical Care*, 2012.

CHAPTER 3: PSYCH-WARD SOJOURN

1. Ontario Consent and Capacity Board Annual Report, 2016/2017, www. ccboard.on.ca/english/publications/documents/annualreport20162017.pdf.

2. Toronto Community Health Profiles, 2012–13 and 2013–14, www.toronto-healthprofiles.ca/a_dataTables.php.

3. Tim Alamenciak and Timothy Appleby, "Charges Laid in Assaults on Mentally Ill in Toronto's Parkdale Neighbourhood," *The Globe and Mail*, May 3, 2011.

4. Parkdale Neighbourhood Land Trust, *No Room for Unkept Promises: Parkdale Rooming Houses Study*, May 2017.

5. Almost 4,000 people apprehended under Ontario's Mental Health Act were dropped off at St. Joe's between 2014 and 2017, 500 more than the second-place hospital, CAMH. (Toronto Police Service statistics released in January 2018, obtained through Access-to-Information request).

6. City of Toronto, Social Housing Waiting List Reports, Q2, 2018.

7. Patricia O'Campo et al, "How did a Housing First intervention improve health and social outcomes among homeless adults with mental illness in Toronto? Two-year outcomes from a randomized trial," *BMJ Open*, September 2016.

CHAPTER 5: WHEN DIAGNOSIS MAKES YOU CRAZY

1. Patrick Barkham, "Green-Haired Turtle that Breathes through Its Genitals Added to Endangered List," *The Guardian*, April 11, 2018.

CHAPTER 7: KNOW THINE ENEMY

1. Madhukar Trivedi, interviewed by the author by phone, October 11, 2016.

2. Paul Kurdyak, interviewed by the author in Toronto, March 30, 2015.

3. Javed Alloo, interviewed by the author in Toronto, September 6, 2016.

4. Ishaq ibn Imran in Andrew Scull, *Madness in Civilization* (Princeton: Princeton University Press, 2015), 56.

5. Andrew Solomon, *The Noonday Demon: An Atlas of Depression* (New York: Scribner, 2001), 31–2.

6. Scull, *Civilization*, 92, 168.

7. National Institute of Mental Health, "Major Depression," www.nimh.nih.gov/health/statistics/major-depression.shtml.

8. Ronald C. Kessler et al, "Lifetime and 12-month Prevalence of DSM-III-R Psychiatric Disorders in the United States," *Arch Gen Psychiatry* (1994).

9. US Centers for Disease Control, "Selected prescription drug classes used in the past 30 days, by sex and age: United States, selected years 1988–1994 through 2011–2014," https://www.cdc.gov/nchs/data/hus/2016/080.pdf.

10. World Health Organization, *Depression and Other Common Mental Disorders: Global Health Estimates*, 2017.

11. WHO, *Depression*, 2017.

12. Sarah Lisanby, interviewed by the author by phone, July 6, 2016.

13. Laura Hirshbein, *American Melancholy: Constructions of Depression in the Twentieth Century* (New Brunswick, NJ: Rutgers University Press, 2009), 59.

CHAPTER 8: CHECKING BOXES

1. *Diagnostic and Statistical Manual of Mental Disorders 5*, "Major Depressive Disorder," (Washington, DC: American Psychiatric Association, 2013).
2. Benoit Mulsant, interviewed by the author by phone, April 23, 2015.
3. Scull, *Civilization*, 392.
4. Elliot Goldner, interviewed by the author by phone, March 20, 2015.
5. Allen Frances, "The New Crisis of Confidence in Psychiatric Diagnosis," *Annals of Internal Medicine* (August 6, 2013), http://annals.org/aim/article /1722526/new-crisis-confidence-psychiatric-diagnosis.
6. Thomas Insel in Scull, *Civilization*, 408.
7. Tom Insel, interviewed by the author by phone, August 23, 2016.

CHAPTER 9: SUICIDE BLUES

1. Jane Pearson, interviewed by the author by phone, July 13, 2016.
2. Jan Neeleman, "Suicide as a Crime in the UK," *Acta Psychiatrica Scandinavica* (1996).
3. Rae Spiwak et al, "Suicide Policy in Canada: Lessons from History," *Canadian Journal of Public Health* (2012).
4. Prakash Behere et al; "Decriminalization of Attempted Suicide Law: Journey of Fifteen Decades," *Indian Journal of Psychiatry* (2015).
5. Jose Manoel Bertolote and Alexandra Fleischman, "Suicide and Psychiatric Diagnosis: A Worldwide Perspective," *World Psychiatry*, October 2002.
6. Maria Oquendo, interviewed by the author by phone, July 13, 2017.
7. Tom Ellis, interviewed by the author by phone, July 26, 2016.
8. World Health Organization, "Suicide: Key Facts," August 24, 2018, www.who.int/news-room/fact-sheets/detail/suicide.
9. Statistics Canada, table 13-10-0392-01, "Deaths and Age-Specific Mortality Rates, by Selected Grouped Causes," www150.statcan.gc.ca/t1/tbl1/en /tv.action?pid=1310039201.
10. You're also more than 63 percent more likely to kill yourself than to die in a car accident and 44 percent more likely to kill yourself than to die of prostate cancer. Statistics Canada, Canadian Vital Statistics, Birth and Death Databases and Appendix II of the publication "Mortality Summary List of Causes," 2012, www150.statcan.gc.ca/n1/pub/84f0209x/2009000/t023-eng.htm.
11. National Violent Death Reporting System, Office of Statistics and Programming, National Center for Injury Prevention and Control, CDC.
12. National Vital Statistics System, National Center for Health Statistics, CDC.
13. J.K. Canner et al, "Emergency Department Visits for Attempted Suicide and Self Harm in the USA: 2006–2013," *Epidemiology and Psychiatric Sciences* (February 2018).

14. National Center for Health Statistics, "Suicide Mortality in the United States, 1999–2017," Centers for Disease Control and Prevention, November 2018, https://www.cdc.gov/nchs/products/databriefs/db330.htm.

15. Sally C. Curtin, Margaret Warner, and Holly Hedegaard, "Increase in Suicide in the United States, 1999–2014," NCHS Data Brief No. 241, April 2016, www.cdc.gov/nchs/products/databriefs/db241.htm.

16. Jane Pearson, interviewed by the author, July 13, 2016.

17. Sarah Lisanby, interviewed by the author, July 6, 2016.

18. Robin Skinner et al, "Suicide in Canada: Is Poisoning Misclassification an Issue?" *Canadian Journal of Psychiatry* (July 2016).

19. Ian R. H. Rockett et al, "Suicide and Unintentional Poisoning Mortality Trends in the United States, 1987–2006: Two Unrelated Phenomena?" *BMC Public Health* (2010).

20. Ian R.H. Rockett et al, "Variable Classification of Drug-Intoxication Suicides across US States: A Partial Artifact of Forensics?" *PLOS One* (August 2015).

21. Skinner et al, "Suicide in Canada."

22. Centers for Disease Control and Prevention, "The Changing Profile of Autopsied Deaths in the United States, 1972–2007," NCHS Data Brief No. 67, August 2011.

23. Rockett et al, "Suicide and Unintentional Poisoning Mortality."

24. Ian Rockett, interviewed by the author by phone, August 2, 2016.

25. Skinner et al, "Suicide in Canada."

26. Rockett et al, "Unintentional Poisoning Mortality."

27. Rockett et al, "Unintentional Poisoning Mortality."

28. Skinner et al, "Suicide in Canada."

29. National Violent Death Reporting System, CDC.

30. 29 percent compared to 51 percent. Ian Rockett et al, "Race/Ethnicity and Potential Suicide Misclassification: Window on a Minority Suicide Paradox?" *BMC Psychiatry* (2010).

31. Rockett et al, "Race/ethnicity and potential suicide misclassification."

32. Rockett, interviewed by the author by phone, August 2, 2016.

33. Michael Peck, interviewed by the author by phone, August 18, 2016.

CHAPTER 11: A PILL-POPPING PARADE

1. Gil Tomer, "Prevailing Against Cost-Leader Competitors in the Pharmaceutical Industry," *Journal of Generic Medicines,* Vol. 5 No. 4 (July 2008).

2. Haiden A. Huskamp, Alisa B. Busch, Marisa E. Domino and Sharon-Lise T. Normand, "Antidepressant Reformulations: Who Uses Them, and What Are the Benefits?" *Health Affairs,* Vol. 28 No. 3 (May/June 2009).

3. Jennifer Tryon and Nick Logan, "Antidepressant Wellbutrin Becomes 'Poor Man's Cocaine' on Toronto Streets," Global News (September 18, 2013).

4. Jakob Nielsen, "Dysregulation of Renal Aquaporins and Epithelial Sodium Channel in Lithium Induced Nephrogenic Diabetes Insipidus," *Seminars i n Nephrology* (May 2008).

5. Ross J. Baldessarini and Leonardo Tondo, "Lithium in Psychiatry," *Revista De Neuro-Psiquiatria* (2013).

6. Martin Alda et al, "Lithium in the Treatment of Bipolar Disorder: Pharmacology and Pharmacogenetics," *Molecular Psychiatry* (2015).

7. Thomas E. Schlaepfer et al, "The Hidden Third: Improving Outcome in Treatment-Resistant Depression," *Journal of Psychopharmacology* (2012); Laura Orsolini et al, "Atypical Antipsychotics in Major Depressive Disorder," *Understanding Depression* (2018).

8. Sven Ulrich, Roland Ricken and Mazda Adli, "Tranylcypromine in Mind (Part I): Review of Pharmacology," *European Neuropsychopharmacology* (April 2017).

9. Roland Ricken, Sven Ulrich, Peter Schlattman and Mazda Adli, "Tranylcypromine in Mind (Part II): Review of Clinical Pharmacology and Meta-analysis of Controlled Studies in Depression," *European Neuropsychopharmacology* (April 2017).

10. Maurizio Fava and A. John Rush, "Current Status of Augmentation and Combination Treatments for Major Depressive Disorder: A Literature Review and a Proposal for a Novel Approach to Improve Practice," *Psychotherapy and Psychosomatics* (2006).

11. Thomas J. Moore, and Donald R. Mattison, "Adult Utilization of Psychiatric Drugs and Differences by Sex, Age, and Race," *JAMA Internal Medicine* (December 2016).

12. Thomas Harr and Lars E. French, "Toxic Epidermal Necrolysis and Stevens-Johnson Syndrome," *Orphanet Journal of Rare Diseases* (2010).

13. Connie Sanchez, Karen E. Asin and Francesca Artigas, "Vortioxetine, a Novel Antidepressant with Multimodal Activity: Review of Preclinical and Clinical Data," *Pharmacology & Therapeutics* (2014).

14. Richard A. Friedman, interviewed by the author by phone, October 19, 2016.

15. They were also more likely to be white or Hispanic, and less likely to be Black, but that could be because of response rates or general likelihood of continued participation: the population was overwhelmingly white all the way through. A. John Rush et al, "Acute and Longer-Term Outcomes in Depressed Outpatients Requiring One or Several Treatment Steps: A STAR*D Report," *American Journal of Psychiatry*, (November 2006).

16. Madhukar Trivedi, interviewed by the author by phone, October 11, 2016.

17. Steven Hyman, interviewed by the author by phone, March 4, 2015.

18. Katelyn R. Keyloun et al, "Adherence and Persistence Across Antidepressant Therapeutic Classes: A Retrospective Claims Analysis Among Insured US Patients with Major Depressive Disorder (MDD)," *CNS Drugs* (April 2017).

19. Elisabeth Y. Bijlsma et al, "Sexual Side Effects of Serotonergic Antidepressants: Mediated by Inhibition of Serotonin on Central Dopamine Release?" *Pharmacology, Biochemistry and Behavior* (October 2013).

20. Arif Khan and Walter Brown, "Antidepressants Versus Placebo in Major Depression: An Overview," *World Psychiatry* (2015).

21. Benoit Mulsant, "Is There a Role for Antidepressant and Antipsychotic Pharmacogenetics in Clinical Practice in 2014?" *Canadian Journal of Psychiatry* (February 2014).

CHAPTER 12: GOOD NOTICING!

1. Beck Institute for Cognitive Behavior Therapy, "History of Cognitive Behavior Therapy," https://beckinstitute.org/about-beck/our-history /history-of-cognitive-therapy/.

2. Steven Hollon et al; "Effect of Cognitive Therapy with Antidepressant Medications vs. Antidepressants Alone on the Rate of Recovery in Major Depressive Disorder," *JAMA Psychiatry* (2014).

3. Christiane Steinert et al; "Relapse Rates after Psychotherapy for Depression—Stable Long-term Effects? A Meta-analysis," *Journal of Affective Disorders* (2014).

4. Mark Olfson and Steven Marcus, "National Patterns in Antidepressant Medication Treatment," *JAMA Psychiatry*, (August 2009).

5. Dennis Greenberger and Christine A. Padesky, authors of the clinically sound, largely helpful bestselling work, *Mind Over Mood: Change How You Feel by Changing the Way You Think* (New York: Guilford Publications, 1995).

6. *Statutory Regulation in Canada.* Canadian Counselling and Psychotherapy Association, 2016.

7. There are guidelines out there: Health Quality Ontario has found evidence for CBT, interpersonal therapy and supportive therapy for depression and anxiety, and recommends publicly covering their provision by non-physicians. (At the time of this writing, they are not.) Health Quality Ontario, "Psychotherapy for Major Depressive Disorder and Generalized Anxiety Disorder: A Health Technology Assessment" and "Psychotherapy for Major Depressive Disorder and Generalized Anxiety Disorder: OHTAC Recommendation," 2017. https://www.hqontario.ca/Portals/0/documents /evidence/reports/hta-psychotherapy-1711.pdf and https://www.hqontario.

ca/Portals/0/documents/evidence/reports/ohtac-recommendations-
psychotherapy-1711-en.pdf.

8.   Michael Schoenbaum, interviewed by the author by phone, July 22, 2016.

CHAPTER 13: ZAPPING, SHOCKING AND BURNING YOUR BRAIN INTO SUBMISSION

1.   Jeff Daskalakis, interviewed by the author in Toronto, August 9, 2016.

2.   Jonathan Downar, Daniel M. Blumberger and Zafiris J. Daskalakis, "Repetitive transcranial magnetic stimulation: an emerging treatment for medication-resistant depression," *CMAJ* (November 2016).

3.   Charles Kellner, interviewed by the author by phone, November 10, 2016.

4.   Georgios Petrides et al; "ECT Remission Rates in Psychotic Versus Nonpsychotic Depressed Patients: A Report from CORE," *The Journal of ECT* (2001); Gerard Gagne et al, "Efficacy of Continuation ECT and Antidepressant Drugs Compared to Long-Term Antidepressants Alone in Depressed Patients," *American Journal of Psychiatry* (2000).

5.   Thomas Insel, interviewed by the author, March 25, 2015.

6.   Sarah Lisanby, "Facebook Q&A on Electroconvulsive Therapy," March 17, 2016.

7.   Charles Kellner et al, "Continuation Electroconvulsive Therapy vs. Pharmacotherapy for Relapse Prevention in Major Depression: A Multisite Study from the Consortium for Research in Electroconvulsive Therapy (CORE)," *Archives of General Psychiatry* (2006).

8.   Darin Dougherty, interviewed by the author by phone, October 13, 2016.

9.   H. Thomas Ballantyne Jr. et al, "Treatment of Psychiatric Illness by Stereotactic Cingulotomy," *Biological Psychiatry* (July 1987).

10. Clemens Janssen et al, "Whole-Body Hyperthermia for the Treatment of Major Depressive Disorder: A Randomized Clinical Trial," *JAMA Psychiatry* (2016).

CHAPTER 14: BRAINIACS

1.   Barbara Lipska, interviewed by the author in Bethesda, MD, July 1, 2016.

2.   Jonathan Sirovatka, interviewed by the author in Bethesda, MD, July 1, 2016.

3.   Melanie Bose, interviewed by the author in Bethesda, MD, July 1, 2016.

4.   Luke Dittrich, *Patient H.M.: A Story of Memory, Madness and Family Secrets* (New York: Random House, 2016).

5.   Kasey N. David et al, "*GAD2* Alternative Transcripts in the Human Prefrontal Cortex, and in Schizophrenia and Affective Disorders," *PlosONE* (February 2016).

6.   Maree Webster, interviewed by the author in Rockville, MD, June 28, 2016.

7.   Gustavo Turecki, interviewed by the author in Montreal, August 8, 2016.

CHAPTER 15: A DRY PHARMA PIPELINE

1. Francisco López-Muñoz and Cecilio Alamo, "Monoaminergic Neurotransmission: The History of the Discovery of Antidepressants from 1950s Until Today," *Current Pharmaceutical Design* (Vol. 15 No. 14, 2009).

2. Steven Hyman, interviewed by the author by phone, March 4, 2015.

3. James W. Murrough and Dennis S. Charney, "Is There Anything Really Novel on the Antidepressant Horizon?" *Current Psychiatry Reports* (December 2012).

4. "Guideline on clinical investigation of medicinal products in the treatment of depression," European Medicines Agency, 2013; Corrado Barbui and Irene Bighelli, "A New Approach to Psychiatric Drug Approval in Europe," *PLOS Medicine* (October 2013).

5. Steven Hyman, interviewed by the author, March 4, 2015.

6. Alison Abbott, "Novartis to Shut Brain Research Facility," *Nature*, December 6, 2011, www.nature.com/news/novartis-to-shut-brain-research-facility-1.9547?nc=1344043518270.

7. Gregers Wegener and Dan Rujescu, "The Current Development of CNS Drug Research," *International Journal of Neuropsychopharmacology* (August 2013).

8. Richard A. Friedman, interviewed by the author by phone, October 19, 2016.

9. Amy E. Sousa, email to the author, January 13, 2017.

10. Steven Danehey, email to the author, November 1, 2016.

11. Mai Tran, email to the author, September 26, 2016.

12. Pamela L. Eisele, email to the author, October 20, 2016.

13. Mark Marmur, email to the author, January 13, 2017.

14. Hyman, interviewed by the author, March 4, 2015.

15. Kenneth Kaitin, interviewed by the author, October 24, 2016.

16. Thomas R. Insel, "The Anatomy of NIMH Funding," www.nimh.nih.gov/funding/funding-strategy-for-research-grants/the-anatomy-of-nimh-funding.shtml.

17. Zul Merali, Keith Gibbs and Keith Busby, "Mental-Health Research Needs More than Private Donations," *The Globe and Mail* (January 29, 2018).

18. Braincanada.ca, accessed Jan. 27, 2018.

CHAPTER 16: OLD ILLNESS, NEW TRICKS—THE ELECTRODE IN YOUR BRAIN

1. Helen Mayberg, interviewed by the author by phone, August 4, 2016.

2. Craig M. Bennett, Abigail A. Baird, Michael B. Miller and George L. Wolford, "Neural Correlates of Interspecies Perspective Taking in the

Post-Mortem Atlantic Salmon: An Argument for Multiple Comparisons Correction," *NeuroImage* (July 2009).

3. Deanna Cole-Benjamin, interviewed by the author in Kingston, ON, November 23, 2016.

4. Takashi Morishita et al, "Deep Brain Stimulation for Treatment-Resistant Depression: Systematic Review of Clinical Outcomes," *Neurotherapeutics* (2014).

5. Justin D. Paquette, email to the author, June 14, 2018.

6. Eric Epperson, email to the author, September 30, 2016.

7. Helen Mayberg, email to the author, January 15, 2019.

8. Darin Dougherty, interviewed by the author by phone, April 20, 2017.

CHAPTER 17: OLD ILLNESS, NEW TRICKS—FROM PSYCHEDELICS TO SMARTPHONES

1. Gerard Sanacora, interviewed by the author in New Haven, June 27, 2016.

2. Benedict Carey, "Fast-Acting Depression Drug, Newly Approved, Could Help Millions," *New York Times*, March 5, 2019.

3. Husseini Manji, interviewed by the author by phone, July 7, 2016.

4. Ella Daly et al, "Efficacy and Safety of Intranasal Esketamine Adjunctive to Oral Antidepressant Therapy in Treatment-Resistant Depression: A Randomized Clinical Trial," *JAMA Psychiatry* (February 2018).

5. Darrick May, interviewed by the author by phone, January 10, 2017.

6. Madhukar Trivedi, interviewed by the author by phone, October 11, 2016.

7. Ken Kaitin, interviewed by the author by phone, October 24, 2016.

8. David Dobbs, "The Smartphone Psychiatrist," *The Atlantic* (July/August 2017).

9. Thomas Insel, interviewed by the author by phone, August 23, 2016.

10. https://mindstronghealth.com/science/ accessed January 16, 2018.

11. John Torous and Laura Weiss Roberts, "Needed Innovation in Digital Health and Smartphone Applications for Mental Health," *JAMA Psychiatry* (May 2017).

12. David Bakker, Nikolaos Kazantzis, Debra Rickwood and Nikki Rickard, "Mental Health Smartphone Apps: Review and Evidence-Based Recommendations for Future Developments," *JMIR Mental Health* (2016).

13. Eric Finzi, interviewed by the author by phone, October 26, 2016.

14. A trial Finzi conducted with Norman Rosenthal, published in 2014, randomized 85 people with major depressive disorder to receive either botulism toxin (onabotulinumtoxinA) or saline injected into their frown muscles. Six weeks after treatment, the study found, subjects' scores on the Montgomery Asberg Depression Rating Scale dropped an average of 47 percent for people who got the botulism and 7 percent for the saline

group. Eric Finzi and Norman Rosenthal, "Treatment of Depression with OnabotulinumtoxinA: A Randomized, Double-Blind, Placebo Controlled Trial," *Journal of Psychiatric Research* (2014). See also Andreas Hennenlotter et al, "The Link Between Facial Feedback and Neural Activity within Central Circuitries of Emotion—New Insights from Botulinum Toxin—Induced Denervation of Frown Muscles," *Cerebral Cortex* (2009); M. Justin Kim et al, "Botulinum Toxin-Induced Facial Muscle Paralysis Affects Amygdala Responses to the Perception of Emotional Expressions: Preliminary Findings from an A-B-A Design," *Biology of Mood and Anxiety Disorders* (2014).

15. Sarah Lisanby, interviewed by the author by phone, January 26, 2017.

CHAPTER 18: STIGMA AND RELATED BULLSHIT

1. https://letstalk.bell.ca/en/.
2. Donna Ferguson in Anna Mehler Paperny, "Mental Illness: How Do I Find Treatment, and What Happens Next?" Globalnews.ca, October 16, 2014.
3. Mary, interviewed by the author in Toronto, August 20, 2016.
4. Claude Di Stasio, interview with the author by phone, August 17, 2016.
5. Karen Cutler, interview with the author by phone, September 22, 2016.
6. Deanna Cole-Benjamin, interview with the author in Kingston, ON, November 23, 2016.
7. Michelle Yan, interviewed by the author in Toronto, December 2, 2016.
8. Hirshbein, *Melancholy.*
9. Gary Newman, text message to the author, October 11, 2017.
10. Lisa, interviewed by the author by phone, August 11, 2016.

CHAPTER 19: THROUGH THE CRACKS

1. Findings and recommendations as a result of the Coroner's Inquest Pursuant to Section 38 of the Coroners Act, [SBC 2007] C 15, into the death of Geisheimer, Brian David; Abdi, Sebastien Pavit; Charles, Sarah Louise, 2015.
2. Alexis Kerr, General Counsel for Fraser Health Authority, "Re: Response to recommendations regarding the Coroner's Inquest into the deaths of: Brian Geisheimer; Sarah Charles; and Sebastian Abdi," September 18, 2018.
3. Paul Kurdyak, interviewed by the author in Toronto, March 25, 2015.
4. Melanie Bose, interviewed by the author in Bethesda, MD, July 1, 2016.
5. Brian K. Ahmedani et al, "Health Care Contacts in the Year before Suicide Death," *Society of General Internal Medicine* (2014).
6. Brian Ahmedani, interviewed by the author by phone, August 1, 2016.
7. zerosuicide.sprc.org.
8. Cathrine Frank, interviewed by the author by phone, November 26, 2018.
9. Jane Pearson, interviewed by the author by phone, July 13, 2016.

10. Mark Olfson, interviewed by the author by phone, September 16, 2016.

11. Javed Alloo, interviewed by the author in Toronto, September 7, 2016.

CHAPTER 20: MENTAL HEALTH IS FOR RICH PEOPLE

1. Centers for Disease Control and Prevention, "Early Release of Estimates from the National Health Interview Survey," January–March 2016; "Pharmacare Now: Prescription Medicine Coverage for All Canadians," *Report of the Standing Committee on Health*, April 2018.

2. Steven C. Marcus, Jeffrey A. Bridge and Mark Olfson, "Payment Source and Emergency Management of Deliberate Self-Harm," *American Journal of Public Health,* Vol. 102 No. 6 (June 2012).

3. Mark Olfson, interviewed by the author by phone, September 16, 2016.

4. Tara Bishop et al; "Acceptance of Insurance by Psychiatrists and the Implications for Access to Mental Health Care," *JAMA Psychiatry* (February 2014).

5. Maria Oquendo, interviewed by the author by phone, July 13, 2017.

6. Tim Bruckner, interviewed by the author in Irvine, CA, July 11, 2016.

7. Joseph H. Puyat, Arminee Kazanjian, Elliot M. Goldner and Hubert Wong, "How Often Do Individuals with Major Depression Receive Minimally Adequate Treatment? A Population-Based, Data Linkage Study," *The Canadian Journal of Psychiatry* (2016).

8. Paul Kurdyak et al, "Universal Coverage without Universal Access: A Study of Psychiatrist Supply and Practice Patterns in Ontario," *Open Medicine* (2014).

9. Paul Kurdyak, interviewed by the author, March 25, 2015.

10. Michael Schoenbaum, interviewed by the author by phone, September 19, 2016.

11. Paul Kurdyak and Sanjeev Sockalingam, "How Canada Fails People with Mental Illness," *Ottawa Citizen* (January 22, 2015).

CHAPTER 21: TRYING TO HEAL THE LITTLEST MINDS

1. Laura Kann et al, "Youth Risk Behavior Surveillance—United States, 2015," *Surveillance Summaries*, US Centers for Disease Control and Prevention, June 10, 2016.

2. Centers for Disease Control and Prevention, Web-based Injury Statistics Query and Reporting System (WISQARS).

3. Arielle Sheftall, interviewed by the author by phone, March 27, 2018.

4. Madelyn Gould, interviewed by the author by phone, March 27, 2018.

5. Jane Pearson, interviewed by the author by phone, July 13, 2016.

6. US Department of Health and Human Services, "Sexual Identity, Sex of Sexual Contacts, and Health-Related Behaviors among Students in Grades

9–12—United States and Selected Sites, 2015," Centers for Disease Control and Prevention, Morbidity and Mortality Weekly Report, August 12, 2016.

7. Ann Haas et al, "Suicide and Suicide Risk in Lesbian, Gay, Bisexual, and Transgender Populations: Review and Recommendations," *Journal of Homosexuality* (January 2011).

8. Haas et al, "Suicide and Suicide Risk."

9. Ann Haas, interviewed by the author by phone, May 18, 2018.

10. Mark L. Hatzenbuehler, Katherine M. Keyes and Deborah S. Hasin, "State-Level Policies and Psychiatric Morbidity in Lesbian, Gay and Bisexual Populations," *American Journal of Public Health* (December 2009).

11. Mark L. Hatzenbeuhler, Katie A. McLaughlin, Katherine M. Keyes and Deborah S. Hasin, "The Impact of Institutional Discrimination on Psychiatric Disorders in Lesbian, Gay and Bisexual Populations: A Prospective Study," *American Journal of Public Health* (March 2010).

12. Ilan H. Meyer, Jessica Dietrich and Sharon Schwartz, "Lifetime Prevalence of Mental Disorders and Suicide Attempts in Diverse Lesbian, Gay, and Bisexual Populations," *American Journal of Public Health* (June 2008).

13. Tarek A. Hammad, "Relationship between Psychotropic Drugs and Pediatric Suicidality," Food and Drug Administration, 2004.

14. Gardiner Harris, "FDA Links Drugs to Being Suicidal," *The New York Times* (September 14, 2004).

15. Christine Y. Lu et al, "Changes in Antidepressant Use by Young People and Suicidal Behavior after FDA Warnings and Media Coverage: Quasi-Experimental Study," *The BMJ* (June 2014); Anne M. Libby, Heather D. Orton and Robert J. Valuck, "Persisting Decline in Depression Treatment after FDA Warnings," *JAMA Psychiatry* (June 2009).

16. "We cannot ignore the weight of these epidemiologic data or the very real possibility that the FDA advisory has unintentionally discouraged depressed patients from seeking treatment and doctors from prescribing antidepressants," psychiatrist Richard A. Friedman wrote, "Antidepressants' Black-Box Warning—10 Years Later," *New England Journal of Medicine* (October 2014).

17. Betsy Kennard, interviewed by the author by phone, March 13, 2018.

18. Marcella, interviewed by the author by phone, October 13, 2016.

CHAPTER 22: "MORE CHILDREN DO NOT HAVE TO DIE"

1. Kerri Cutfeet, interviewed by the author by phone, August 12, 2017.

2. Michael Kirlew, Affidavit before the Canadian Human Rights Tribunal; January 27, 2017.

3. Alvin Fiddler, "Re: Preventable Deaths of Our Youth," email to Prime Minister Justin Trudeau, January 18, 2017. Exhibit B referred to in the affidavit of Dr. Michael Kirlew, Canada Human Rights Tribunal, January 27, 2017.

4. Joshua Frogg, interviewed by the author by phone, July 12, 2017.

5. Michael Kirlew; Affidavit, January 27, 2017.

6. US Centers for Disease Control Web-based Injury Statistics Query and Reporting System Database; accessed July 27–29, 2017.

7. Caroline Jiang et al. "Racial and Gender Disparities in Suicide among Young Adults Aged 18–24: United States, 2009–2013," Centers for Disease Control and Prevention, September 2015.

8. https://wemattercampaign.org/

9. Gordon Poschwatta, interviewed by the author by phone, November 3, 2016.

10. Henry Harder, interviewed by the author by phone, October 28, 2016.

11. Eva Serhal et al, "Implementation and Utilisation of Telepsychiatry in Ontario: A Population-Based Study," *Canadian Journal of Psychiatry*, 2017.

12. Cindy Hardy, interviewed by the author by phone, October 20, 2016.

13. Michael Kirlew, interviewed by the author by phone, July 31, 2017.

CHAPTER 23: RACE AS BARRIER

1. Hector M. Gonzalez, "Depression Care in the United States: Too Little for Too Few," *Archives of General Psychiatry* (2010).

2. Leopoldo Cabassa et al, "Latino Adults' Access to Mental Health Care: A Review of Epidemiological Studies," *Administration and Policy in Mental Health* (2006).

3. Carrie Farmer Teh et al, "Predictors of Adequate Depression Treatment among Medicaid-Enrolled Adults," *Health Services Research* (February 2010).

4. Rudayna Bahubeshi, "Canada: Let's Really Talk about Mental Illness and Who's Most Vulnerable," CBC.ca (October 2, 2017).

5. Rheeda Walker, interviewed by the author by phone, November 9, 2016.

6. Gursharan Virdee, interviewed by the author by phone, May 9, 2018.

7. Napoleon Harrington, interviewed by the author by phone, March 24, 2018.

8. Jasmin Pierre, interviewed by the author by phone, July 29, 2016.

9. Maria Chiu et al, "Ethnic Differences in Mental Illness Severity: A Population-Based Study of Chinese and South Asian Patients in Ontario, Canada," *J Clin Psychiatry* (2016).

10. Maria Chiu, interviewed by the author by phone, October 4, 2016.

11. Maria Chiu et al, "Postdischarge Service Utilisation and Outcomes among Chinese and South Asian Psychiatric Inpatients in Ontario, Canada: A Population-Based Cohort Study," *BMJ Open* (2018).

12. Meri Nana-Ama Danquah, *Willow Weep for Me* (New York: W.W. Norton & Company, 1998), 224.

CHAPTER 24: WHO YOU GONNA CALL?

1. Susan Stefan, interviewed by the author by phone, November 3, 2016.
2. Ontario Human Rights Commission, *A Collective Impact*, December 10, 2018.
3. Daryl Kramp, *Economics of Policing: Report of the Standing Committee on Public Safety and National Security*, May 2014, 41st Parliament, Second Session.
4. Anna Mehler Paperny, "Outgoing Toronto Police Services Board Chair Alok Mukherjee on Reimagining Toronto Cops," Globalnews.ca, June 18, 2015.
5. Anna Mehler Paperny, "Taser Files: What We Found in 594 Pages of Taser Incident Reports," Global News, July 7, 2015.
6. Joel Dvoskin, interviewed by the author by phone, November 7, 2016.
7. Peter Eisler, Jason Szep, Tim Reid and Grant Smith, "Shock Tactics," Reuters, August 22, 2017.
8. Vincent Beasley, interviewed by the author by phone, November 6, 2017.
9. Wendy Gillis, "Toronto Police Curb Disclosure of Suicide Attempts to US Border Police," *Toronto Star,* August 17, 2015.
10. Scott Gilbert, interviewed by the author in Toronto, January 12, 2018.

CHAPTER 25: HOW TO TALK ABOUT WHAT WE TALK ABOUT WHEN WE TALK ABOUT WANTING TO DIE

1. David Jobes, interviewed by the author by phone, August 1, 2016.
2. Yunqiao Wang et al, "Clinician Prediction of Future Suicide Attempts: A Longitudinal Study," *The Canadian Journal of Psychiatry,* April 2016.
3. Yunqiao Wang, interviewed by the author by phone, July 21, 2016.
4. Aaron T. Beck and Maria Kovacs, "Assessment of Suicidal Intention: The Scale for Suicide Ideation," *Journal of Consulting and Clinical Psychology* (1979).
5. Paul Kurdyak, interviewed by the author in Toronto, March 30, 2015.
6. Javed Alloo, interviewed by the author in Toronto, September 7, 2016.
7. Sarah Lisanby, interviewed by the author by phone, July 6, 2016.
8. Maria Oquendo, interviewed by the author by phone, July 13, 2017.
9. Marcel Adam Just et al; "Machine Learning of Neural Representations of Suicide and Emotion Concepts Identifies Suicidal Youth," *Nature Human Behaviour* (2017).
10. Tom Ellis, interviewed by the author by phone, July 26, 2016.
11. Brian Ahmedani, interviewed by the author by phone, August 1, 2016.
12. Kurt Kroenke, Robert L. Spitzer and Janet B.W. Williams, "The PHQ-9: Validity of a Brief Depression Severity Measure," *Journal of General Internal Medicine,* September 2001.

13. Madelyn Gould et al, "Newspaper Coverage of Suicide and Initiation of Suicide Clusters in Teenagers in the USA, 1988–96: A Retrospective, Population-Based, Case-Control Study," *Lancet Psychiatry* (2014).

14. Madelyn Gould, interviewed by the author by phone, March 27, 2018.

15. David A. Jobes et al, "The Kurt Cobain Suicide Crisis: Perspectives from Research, Public Health, and the News Media," *Suicide and Life-Threatening Behaviour* (Fall 1996).

16. Stephanie Leon et al; "Media Coverage of Youth Suicides and Its Impact on Paediatric Mental Health Emergency Department Presentations," *Healthcare Policy*, 2014.

17. Mario Cappelli, interviewed by the author by phone, October 31, 2017.

18. Solomon, *Noonday Demon*, 251.

CHAPTER 26: CERTIFIABLE

1. E. Fuller Torrey, *American Psychosis: How the Federal Government Destroyed the Mental Illness Treatment System* (New York: Oxford University Press, 2014), 93.

2. Claims History Database, Registered Persons Dabatase, Ontario Mental Health Reporting System, obtained from Ontario Ministry of Health and Long-Term Care, November 2, 2017, through media request. Data extracted March 2017 and November 2017.

3. The number of visits by girls under eighteen being kept on two-week certifications more than tripled; the number of month-long stays increased sixfold (although the starting number was small). And in almost 90 percent of cases these girls are being held to protect themselves from themselves. Ontario Ministry of Health and Long-Term Care, November 2017.

4. Integrated Analytics: Hospital, Diagnostics Workforce Branch, Health Sector Information, Analysis and Reporting Division, obtained from British Columbia Ministry of Mental Health and Addictions, October 23, 2017, through media request.

5. Statistics obtained from Alberta Health Services November 15, 2017, through media request. I was obliged to get involuntary hospitalization data for Saskatchewan at the health region level. The number of compulsory hospital admissions in Saskatoon Health Region increased 88 percent between 2010 and 2016, and the number of certificates issued for involuntary ECT doubled during that time, according to statistics from the health region obtained November 28, 2017, through access-to-information request. The number of people put on community treatment orders province-wide more than tripled between 2013–14 and 2016–17, according to Saskatchewan government statistics obtained December 27, 2017, through access-to-information request.

6. Hans Joachim Salize et al, "Compulsory Admission and Involuntary Treatment of Mentally Ill Patients—Legislation and Practice in EU-Member States," European Commission Health & Consumer Protection Directorate-General, 2002.

7. Hans Joachim Salize et al, "Compulsory Admission."

8. Patrick Keown et al, "Rates of Voluntary and Compulsory Psychiatric In-Patient Treatment in England: An Ecological Study Investigating Associations with Deprivation and Demographics," *The British Journal of Psychiatry* (2016).

9. Scott Weich et al, "Variation in Compulsory Psychiatric Inpatient Admission in England: A Cross-Classifed, Multilevel Analysis," *Lancet Psychiatry* (2017).

10. Black people made up 13 percent of the Toronto residents on CTOs between 2005–06 and 2010–11 despite comprising about 7 percent of the population. R.A. Malatest and Associates Ltd., Legislated Review of Community Treatment Orders, May 2012.

11. Jorun Rugkasa, "Why We Need to Understand Service Variation in Compulsion," *Lancet Psychiatry*, 2017.

12. Richard O'Reilly, interviewed by the author by phone, February 29, 2016.

13. Wendy Glauser, "Scrubbed: Ontario Emergency Room Chief Faces Questions about Failing to Hire Any Female Doctors in 16 Years," *The Globe and Mail*, December 16, 2018.

14. Anita Szigeti, interviewed by the author by phone, July 8, 2017.

15. Treatment Advocacy Center, Browse By State, www.treatmentadvocacycenter .org/browse-by-state.

16. Jay Chalke, *Committed to Change: Protecting the Rights of Involuntary Patients under the Mental Health Act*, Special Report No. 42, March 2019.

17. Jeffrey Swanson, interviewed by the author by phone, July 18, 2016.

18. Deanna Cole-Benjamin, interviewed by the author in Kingston, ON, November 23, 2016.

19. Leslie, interviewed by the author by phone, August 5, 2016.

20. Cindy, interviewed by the author by phone, October 9, 2016.

21. Andrew Lustig, interviewed by the author in Toronto, July 12, 2017.

22. Joel Dvoskin, interviewed by the author by phone, November 7, 2016.

23. E. Fuller Torrey, interviewed by the author in Kensington, MD, June 28, 2016.

24. Eight of 12 studies in a broad review of the evidence for community treatment orders found they reduced hospital readmission. But methodologies varied; the argument could be made that someone's improvement was due to access to intervention, rather than the compulsion itself. Outcomes are better for people who are on CTOs for a longer period of time but that could be because people are kept on the CTO longer explicitly

because they're doing well. And hospitalization outcome differences between people on orders and off them were negligible in the few studies that were randomized. "The lack of evidence for patient benefit, particularly when combined with restrictions to personal liberty, is striking and needs to be taken seriously," the study's authors write. "Clinicians have a duty to provide their patients with treatment in the least restrictive environment." Jorun Rugkasa, John Dawson and Tom Burns, "CTOs: What Is the State of the Evidence?" *Social Psychiatry and Psychiatric Epidemiology* (February 2014).

25. Statistics obtained through media request from Ontario's Office of the Chief Coroner, October 18, 2017.
26. Erin Hawkes, "Medicate me, even when I refuse," *Huffington Post,* 2013.
27. Daryl Geisheimer, interviewed by the author by phone, September 8, 2017.
28. Mark Lukach, *My Lovely Wife in the Psych Ward* (New York: HarperCollins, 2017).

CHAPTER 27: TRUST ISSUES

1. Laney, interviewed by the author by phone, August 5, 2016.
2. "The Bonnie Burstow Scholarship in Antipsychiatry," OISE, University of Toronto, November 16, 2016, www.oise.utoronto.ca/oise/News/Bonnie _Burstow_Scholarship.html.
3. Bonnie Burstow, interviewed by the author by phone, May 19, 2017.
4. Husseini Manji, interviewed by the author by phone, July 7, 2016.
5. Gary Greenberg, *Manufacturing Depression* (London: Bloomsbury Publishing, 2010), 334.
6. Gary Greenberg, interviewed by the author by phone, April 18, 2017.
7. Paul Kurdyak, interviewed by the author, March 30, 2015.
8. Patrick, interviewed by the author in Toronto, June 24, 2016.
9. Ethan McIlhenny et al, "Methodology for and the Determination of the Major Constituents and Metabolites of the Amazonian Botanical Medicine Ayahuasca in Human Urine," *Biomedical Chromatography,* November 2010.

CHAPTER 28: FIRST PERSON AFTERWORD

1. Andrew Solomon, interviewed by the author in New York City, October 18, 2016.
2. Helen Mayberg, interviewed by the author, August 4, 2016.

Index